LOSING 50 AFTER 50

RECLAIM YOUR HEALTH AND GET YOUR BODY BACK!

BY KATIE OWEN

For more information, email: hello@losing50after50.com.

ISBN: 979-8-9888449-0-7 (print)

ISBN: 979-8-9888449-1-4 (ebook)

GET YOUR FREE GIFT!

To reclaim your health and get your body back faster, download and use the *Losing 50 After 50 Workbook.* The workbook is designed with you in mind, and it's one place for all your notes! Journal the insights you receive while reading the incredible stories of victory from multiple weight loss journeys. Record personal reasons for embarking on your own weight loss journey. Document the steps you're willing to take and create your own plan. Set goals and track your progress!

You can get a copy by visiting:

Losing50After50.com

DEDICATION

This book is dedicated to Bill, my handsome husband. Without his support, this book wouldn't exist. Because of his support, many lives will be positively impacted!

CONTENTS

FOREWORD

It has been my distinguished honor to know and serve Katie along with her family for the better part of a decade and a half. Not only is she a knowledgeable resource in the literary journey you are about to embark on, but she is an exceptional human being. She is a thriving entrepreneur, a savvy, supportive wife to her husband Bill, and a stand-out mother to her two kids: Alison and Andrew. Katie is as honest and as hard-working as they come.

You see, what I have learned in my almost 20 years of private practice is that there is no magic formula; no pill, potion, or lotion will give you any sort of advantage over the next person. A lesson that many Americans are currently learning the hard way. Don't believe me? Well then, how would you explain a multi-billion-dollar supplement industry in a country that has an obesity rate that exceeds 40%? How would you also explain a country, the United States, that spends more on health care than any other nation in the world but is ranked **last** in comparison to other industrialized countries such as the United Kingdom, Switzerland, Sweden, Australia, and even Costa Rica? Yes, you read that correctly! The truth is that most people spend more time on their cell phones in a single year than they will on their own health in a lifetime.

With overwhelming statistics like these, what makes Katie's *Losing 50* After *50* any different from something you could pick up at Barnes and Noble or on Amazon? One word...**GRIT!** Katie has it! She will take you on a brilliantly simplistic voyage to regaining your health. She is not only the author of the book, but Katie truly lives the principles she shares in the pages ahead. I've seen her transformation with my own eyes. I've watched the pounds come off. I've witnessed her confidence soar and her energy levels skyrocket. I've had the pleasure of witnessing what it's done for her marriage and her relationship with her kids.

So, the question I leave you with is this. Are you worth it? Answer out loud. Are you worth it?! Is a higher quality of life worth it? Is your spouse worth it? Are your kids worth it? Are your grandkids worth it? Are the life experiences you could have as a slimmer, more energized **YOU** worth it? If the answer is yes, then turn the page, buckle up, and prepare to change your life... **you deserve it!!**

Mark W. Taylor, D.C.

INTRODUCTION

I hate diets. I hate diet books.

However, I figured out how to lose 50 pounds. And I love books that inspire me to become better.

So, I have done the unimaginable. I have written a book about dieting. Well, not really a diet, but a lifestyle I created that included radically changing the food I ate. Some call it a diet, and others call it a lifestyle. I'm just excited to have finally figured out how to lose the 50 extra pounds that have been plaguing me for decades. When I began losing weight, these questions soon followed: "How are you doing it?" and "Can you share your smoothie recipes with me?"

Wanting to help my friends, I documented each of my smoothie recipes and began sharing them. The problem was that most people weren't willing or able to drink three smoothies a day to lose weight. It's harsh, I get it. It worked for me, but it won't work for everyone.

As I was having increased success in losing weight, my friends and clients began to tell me their stories of weight loss and how they did it. While there are similarities between "how we did it", there are differences. It occurred to me that it would benefit my friends and family to hear multiple stories of how different people have been successful with losing 50 or more pounds, most of them after the age of 50.

What's so special about losing weight after age 50?

As I've shared with people about the book I'm writing, they inevitably ask the question, "What's so special about losing weight after age 50?" In my opinion, the ability to lose weight after 40 was tough. Now, after age 50, it seemed impossible. The metabolism slows down, the body feels more set in its ways, and the willpower to make it happen is almost non-existent. I used to ruminate aloud, "What age do I have to be to stop caring about my weight and how I look?" I seriously wanted just to give up and accept my larger size. Between not feeling that I could lose the extra weight and not wanting to do the work to make it happen, I was looking for someone to give me a pass. Thankfully, I never fully gave up; finally, I found my personal low place and began the work to climb out of what felt like an abyss.

My goal is to inspire you through stories and strategies. My sincere hope is that you will keep an open mind as you read this book and make the decision to lose your extra weight. More than a system or plan, you need to decide that you have had enough of being overweight and choose something better for yourself. Once the decision is made, create a personalized plan that will work for you. You know your body better than anyone else. Decide what you're willing to do and do it!

I was listening to a podcast recently. The host was talking about how people ask for a list of steps to begin something new. He said that people are always wanting to be told how to do something and then be given a plan of action. He shared that people don't need a plan of action; they simply need to decide to *do* something about their current situation. He likened it to holding a snake. If you are holding a snake, you don't ask someone else what steps you should take to get rid of it. You make the decision to get rid of the snake, and you figure out how to do it! Immediately!

So, make the decision to reclaim your health and get your body back!

What This Book Is

This book is a collection of stories from real people who have lost 50 or more pounds, most of them after age 50. I interviewed each person profiled and asked a series of questions about their weight loss journey. I created a list of the important things that people would likely want to know. I posted the initial list on social media and asked my friends what questions they would like me to add, and I received great feedback! You will notice that I asked everyone the same questions. Here they are:

List of Questions

- How old were you when you began your weight loss journey?
- How tall are you and what was your starting and ending weight?
- How long did it take you to lose your weight?
- Why did you begin? What prompted you to begin? And why now, after 50 years?
- Have you dieted before (prior to the weight loss we are discussing)? What did you do then vs. now?
- Did you follow a specific program?
- What did you do for exercise?
- What foods did you eat?
- What foods did you stay away from?
- Are there any foods you have absolutely eliminated?
- Did you eat meat? Which ones?
- Did you use any apps like MyFitnessPal or FitBit?
- What are your favorite snacks?
- What are your favorite recipes?
- Did you drink alcohol during your journey?
- Are you drinking alcohol now?
- How does your day-to-day look during maintenance?
- How do you manage holidays, eating out, celebrations, etc.?
- How did you deal with your weight loss during illness?

- How did you get through plateaus?
- How did you catch yourself before it felt like it was "too late" or you've "fallen off the wagon"?
- How did you manage your family and friends and their lack of support?
- How did you handle cooking for your family when you ate foods different from theirs?
- What did you learn late in your journey that you wish you had known at the beginning?
- Did you have any medication or health changes because of your weight loss?
- What is your internal conversation around your weight loss journey?
- What do you say to yourself: 1) after a day of poor eating; 2) when your weight goes up; 3) when you are tempted?
- What are your weight loss hacks?
- What's the best part of losing weight?

You'll notice that the people I interviewed have strong opinions about what did and didn't work for them. Some approaches taken were diametrically opposed to one another. Instead of discounting conflicting alternatives or being confused as to which route you should take, consider which path resonates with you more and choose that way. As one of my interviewees said, "You do you." What's important is for you to draw a line in the sand and move forward! Make the decision to reclaim your health. Create a plan that will work for you. And enjoy everything that comes with a slimmer, more energetic body!

What This Book Is Not

This book is not a specific program or list of steps. It is not one person's story; it is the story of many people. Based on feedback received through social media, I also interviewed a Medical Doctor, a Registered and Licensed Dietician (specializing in weight management and diabetes), and a previous professional weight loss coach.

Please note that I am not a medical professional. This book does not give nutritional or medical advice. I am simply sharing what I and others have done to reclaim our health and get our bodies back after years of being overweight. It is always wise to seek medical advice from a doctor or professional you trust before attempting anything new that can affect your health.

My challenge for you is to look for one thing you can implement from each person's story. Is there a weight loss hack, recipe, or workout you are willing to try? I incorporated many of the things I learned into my daily life, and they have been helpful in different ways. I will reveal my new habits at the end of the book. I do not want to influence your choices of what you are willing to put in motion for yourself.

In the world of sales, there's a useful phrase that goes like this, "Have you heard enough to make a decision?" I don't know if this phrase was coined by Grant Cardone, but he teaches it, and I've definitely learned it from him. The idea behind the question is to find out if your prospect is ready to move forward with the sale. The sale *I'm* attempting to make with this book is for you to choose health. I want this book to impact your life. Throughout this book, I'm going to ask you if you've heard enough to decide in favor of your health. Then I'm going to encourage you to: make the decision, create your plan, and get your body back!

To reclaim your health and get your body back faster, download and use the free resource *Losing 50 After 50 Workbook*. You can download the workbook at Losing50After50.com. The workbook is designed with you in mind, and it's one place for all your notes! Journal the insights you receive while reading the incredible stories of victory from multiple weight loss journeys. Record personal reasons for embarking on your own weight loss journey. Document the steps you're willing to take and create your own plan. Set goals and track your progress!

For the free workbook and additional resources, please visit Losing50After50.com. I would love the opportunity to cheer you on and hear about your successes! You can also leave me a helpful book review on my website.

One last thing before we jump in... This book was written 100% by me, Katie Owen (a human), not by Artificial Intelligence or Chat GPT. The foreword was written by Mark W. Taylor, D.C. (also a human). With the growing popularity of AI-generated content, I felt it was important to let you know that no AI was used in the creation or editing of this book.

Now let's dive in together!

CHAPTER 1
KATIE'S STORY

I am 5'8" tall and my highest documented weight was 209 pounds. I began my weight loss journey at age 50, and it took me one year to lose 50 pounds, with my lowest weight coming in at 156 pounds. Here is my story of how I did it.

Don't post that photo! It was March 2022, and my friends and I had just enjoyed a wonderful birthday brunch to celebrate our friend Tracy's birthday. As always, we took a group photo to commemorate the occasion. Since the photo was taken with my phone, it was up to me to forward it to the group. I sent it but then regretted it immediately. I quickly followed up with a text asking them not to post the picture on social media.

As I was assessing the picture and why I looked so heavy, I told myself it was the dress. My husband never liked that dress anyway, so why did I choose to wear it to the birthday brunch? Honestly, I was trying to wear something cute and different because all my large clothes were frumpy and not attractive. After blaming the dress, I also blamed my location in a picture. You're supposed to put the skinny girls at the ends and in front for the picture and hide behind them, with only your pretty face and smile showing. Lastly, I blamed the style of the dress. I should not be wearing a dress with no sleeves. I wore a long black sweater to cover my large arms, but it wasn't helping. The reality was that I was heavy, and it showed in pictures. Period.

This wasn't the first time I looked heavy in a picture. But it was the first time I asked others not to post an otherwise great picture of our group (at least that I could remember). In fact, I was so used to being heavy that I told myself I had to embrace how I looked in pictures. I couldn't go through life deleting pictures of family and friends. I didn't like being overweight, but unless I chose to lose the weight, I had to own it.

Many people asked me what led to the point where I was willing to do whatever it took to lose weight. Prior to my second child, Andrew (now 17 as of the writing of this book), I weighed 150 pounds, and I gained 50 pounds during his pregnancy. The extra weight from my second pregnancy didn't come off so easily. I believe at one point, I was down to 165 pounds, but that was six years after I had Andrew.

I remember being at a neighborhood ladies' get-together and speaking to one of the gals who had lost her pregnancy weight quickly (in my opinion). I said, "Wow! You look great! Have you lost all your baby weight?" She answered, "I should hope so, it's been four months." I thought to myself, it's been four years since my last child was born, and I haven't lost the weight.

Over the years, the weight packed on. I would lose 10-15 pounds on different diets and twenty pounds after doing a 28-day water fast to detox, but the weight would always come back. I had the following commentaries going through my head:

- "It doesn't matter what I eat. I can't lose weight."
- "I just want to eat (fill in the blank). I don't care if I gain weight."
- "I'm over 40, and my metabolism has slowed down."
- "I'm over 50. When can I stop worrying about how I look?"
- "I'm not that heavy. Plenty of people would love to be my weight."

Oh, the lies we tell ourselves!

I am a licensed health and life insurance agent. I help overwhelmed Medicare-eligible people successfully navigate the enrollment process. As I work with my clients, I request a list of their prescription medications so that I can help them find the best drug insurance plan. It never fails: my clients who have a number of medications also have many health issues, whereas my clients who take no medications generally like to share that they are active and eat well. Overall, they also weigh less than my clients, who have many health issues. The truth is, I am motivated by my unhealthy clients to get healthy. At age 50, I was a mere 15 years away from being eligible for Medicare (which begins at age 65). I had a choice. Did I want to be on multiple medications and battle health issues, or did I want to be medication-free and healthy? It's a stark choice that's in my face every day.

Another contributing factor to my willingness to lose weight occurred in August 2021. I broke the fifth metatarsal bone in my left foot. With no significant healing after 18 weeks, I had a titanium screw surgically inserted into my left foot in December 2021. Including post-op, I wore a walking boot for the better part of 30 weeks. *Insert eyeroll and groan here.*

At about six weeks post-op, I hit another low when I went for my annual physical. Did you know that when you go for a physical, you do not have to be weighed if you don't want to be? Or if you are weighed, you can turn your back to the scale and not see your weight? Just tell the nurse you don't want to be told your weight. They smile and record it, then walk you to your room. I had been doing this little practice for years. Remember, I was telling myself there was nothing I could do about my high weight. Let's be honest, I was playing the victim. In my victim mindset, I didn't want to know how much I weighed because then, it wasn't real. So, there I was at my annual physical, and my doctor said, "Wow! 209 pounds! That's a new high for you!" I was thinking, are you kidding me? Just five minutes earlier, I turned my back to the scale because I didn't want to know my weight! I pointed to my walking boot and said, "I weighed with my boot on." She said, "Well, that accounts for a few pounds. You should really work on losing some weight." I wanted to scream that if I didn't have a broken foot, I could work out, and I wouldn't be this heavy! Instead, I politely smiled and agreed.

In March 2022, I attended the 10X GrowthCon business conference put on by Grant Cardone. At this annual event, he brings successful people from all walks of life onto his stage to tell their "come up" stories. As a business owner, I feel it's important to constantly learn and grow. My goals are to be the best insurance agent for my clients, to lead my team well and build a successful insurance agency. Since I've never built a large agency, I need to learn from others who have built remarkably successful businesses. Therefore, I submitted myself to regular teaching and mentoring from successful people.

During this conference, I was inspired to put my money where my mouth is and make a financial investment in my business. I invested in a few advantageous programs and took my personal and business growth to a whole new level. I learned the things I needed to do as a business owner to help my team and move my business forward, but I couldn't just work on my business and not work on myself. Everything affects everything else. If I didn't feel good about myself, I wasn't going to feel good about building my business and doing the things that needed to be done. I made the investment in myself; it was important to get this right.

One of the things I invested in during this conference was performing a genetic test offered by 10X Health System. The test looks for breaks in our genes. Certain gene breaks can be supplemented by vitamins. Other people who had taken the test and begun the supplementation were talking about how good they felt and their increased energy. I wanted to feel better, so I signed up, tested my whole family, and began taking the recommended vitamin supplements. I began feeling better, and my energy and stamina improved. To complete your own gene testing, visit 10XHealthSystem.com to learn more.

At 12 weeks post-op, I was fully released to walk to my heart's content. Believing that exercise alone was the answer to my high weight, I quickly worked up to five miles per day, 6-7 days per week. It felt so good to be moving again, but I was not losing the weight. March, April, and May went by, and I wasn't making much progress at all.

During my daily walks, I would often run into other ladies (whom I'd known for years) who were also walking for exercise. One of them, Patty, had lost 87 pounds (at that point). She looked amazing, and I was intrigued. She said she changed the food she ate and began walking every morning. Other than that, she hadn't done anything unique or bizarre to lose so much weight. Her story is later in this book. I was so impressed by Patty's success; I knew I should at least try.

I began thinking about the times in my life when I had successfully lost weight. I once lost weight eating low carb/high protein, but that was in my twenties, and I was never able to lose weight again with that approach. I also tried the Daniel Diet, but I didn't have enough motivation to stick with it. I once tried the Blood Type Diet, but that didn't work either. I also tried a 10-day diet with extremely specific foods. For the first five days, I had to eat considerable amounts of fruit. I loved the first half of that diet because I love fruit. But then the next five days, I had to eat vegetables. I'm fine with vegetables in a smoothie, but I'm not excited to eat a bunch of raw vegetables. I mentioned my water fast earlier; in 2018, I did a 28-day water fast and lost around twenty pounds. The only problem was that the weight came back once I began eating food again. Go figure! But moving on...

First, I made the decision to *lose* the weight. Second, I created my plan based on what I was willing to *do*.

I wanted to do something that was like water fasting but had more calories and included protein. I really enjoy smoothies, and so much nutrition can be packed into them. I also had to create a plan that I could stick with day after day, week after week, and month after month. I desperately wanted my body back and was willing to do anything to make it happen for as long as necessary. So, I began a smoothie fast. I had already been doing my breakfast smoothie for years. This smoothie had such amazing ingredients that my chiropractor (Mark W. Taylor, D.C.) called it a powerhouse smoothie. I make all my smoothies in a Vitamix blender (I've owned my Vitamix blender since 1994, and it works really well).

Below are my smoothie recipes. As you review them, don't get stuck if there's an ingredient you don't like. Create a variation you're willing to do if you enjoy smoothies!

Breakfast "Powerhouse" Smoothie

Organic Coconut Water (12 ounces)

Organic Spring Mix Lettuce (2 handfuls)

Organic Garden of Life – Chocolate Protein (1 scoop)

Organic Ground Chia Seeds (1 tablespoon)

Organic Cocoa Powder (1 tablespoon)

Organic Chlorella Powder (1 teaspoon to start, work up to 1 tablespoon)

Wyman's Triple Berry Blend (frozen raspberries, blueberries & blackberries) (1/2 to 1 cup)

Organic Sprouts (sproutpeople.org) (1 handful; optional, I grow my own.) (I prefer the "Italian" blend of seeds.)

Ice Cubes (6)

Add all ingredients into blender. Blend on high for 30 seconds. Remove blender from base, shake ingredients, return to base, and blend on high again for 30 seconds.

Makes a 20 oz smoothie. Pour into cup and use large straw (the smoothie is thick).

Next, I had to create a lunchtime smoothie. I did a few different iterations and produced a super delicious lunch smoothie.

Lunch Smoothie

Organic Coconut Water (12 ounces)

Organic Spring Mix Lettuce (2 handfuls)

Organic Garden of Life – Vanilla Protein (1 scoop)

Organic Celery (2 medium-length stalks)

Apple – (half an apple)

Organic Frozen Peaches (4-5 slices)

Organic Frozen Dark Sweet Cherries (8-10 cherries)

Ice Cubes (6)

Add all ingredients into blender. Blend on high for 30 seconds. Remove blender from base, shake ingredients, return to base, and blend on high again for 30 seconds.

Makes a 28 oz smoothie. Pour into cup and use large straw (the smoothie is thick).

Finally, I had to develop a dinnertime smoothie. For some reason, I drink this one the fastest.

Dinner Smoothie

Organic Coconut Water (12 ounces)

Organic Spring Mix Lettuce (2 handfuls)

Organic Garden of Life – Vanilla Protein (1 scoop)

Organic Cucumber (1/3 of a cucumber)

Organic Avocado (1/2 of an avocado)

Organic (fresh-squeezed) Lime Juice (1-2 ounces of fresh lime juice)

Ice Cubes (6)

Add all ingredients into blender. Blend on high for 30 seconds. Remove blender from base, shake ingredients, return to base, and blend on high again for 30 seconds.

Makes a 20 oz smoothie. Pour into cup and use large straw (the smoothie is thick).

Weigh yourself every day. Every morning, I get up and use the bathroom (or "freshen up," as my father likes to say). Before drinking or eating anything, I weigh myself with no clothes except my underwear. I don't put major emphasis on my weight unless it goes down. If it goes up, I say to myself, "Hmm, that's interesting," or "That's okay." When it goes down, I throw my arms in the air in a high "V" and pump them a few times (yes,

I was a cheerleader in high school). I tell myself, "Way to go! You rock!" One benefit of weighing yourself daily is to see the constant fluctuation, WHICH IS COMPLETELY NORMAL.

Through the process of interviewing people, I learned that our bodies need to adjust to our new lower weight before we lose more. This can look like a plateau or like this: 166, 167, 166.5, 168, 170, 167.5, 171, 169.5, etc. The benefit of weighing daily is to experience the new low, to watch the weight go up but then also come back down. When I only weighed once a week (on previous diets), and I did not appear to be making progress week after week, I felt discouraged for the next seven days, and it was harder to stay motivated.

Claim your new lowest weight. It is so exhausting telling people that I've lost 35 pounds, now 34, now 33, now 33.5, now 32, now 30, now 32.5, now 29, now 30.5... Oh my gosh, just stop!!! Claim your new lowest weight and be done with it. I also don't claim ½ pounds. I claim the full pound lost. So, when I weighed 165.5 pounds, I triumphantly said I had lost 44 pounds. I have a friend whose scale tracks pounds and ounces. She would tell me her new weight every day, and it was up two ounces or down four ounces from the day before. That was exhausting. Just claim your new lowest weight at the full pound mark and move on! Since our weight fluctuates up and down during the weight loss journey, I don't think it's helpful to focus on anything other than your new lowest weight.

As I was weighing myself daily, I noticed that my weight would drop two pounds, then go up a pound or three, but then it would come back down again. It's as if my body would try out a new, lower weight but then say, "Nope! That's too low; let's go up again before we settle on that lower weight." My massage therapist, Leisa Pimm, likens this phenomenon to a stand-off. It's our bodies saying, "Are you going to keep feeding me? If so, I'll give up more weight. If not, I won't budge from this number." I also noticed that my clothes would feel loose before my weight dropped. I'm still bewildered by the fact that we often lose inches before pounds.

After about three months of drinking mostly smoothies, I began adding solid food back into my diet. I chose healthy foods that I enjoy eating. It's important to eat foods you enjoy instead of foods "they" say you should eat; I ate all kinds of meats (steak, chicken, turkey) and salmon. For a side dish, I would have Brussels sprouts, steamed squash, or green beans. For snacks, I enjoyed eating pumpkin seeds and fruit (dates, prunes, dried apricots, red seedless grapes, or an apple).

From time to time, I also chose higher-calorie foods that were not as healthy (my vices are tortilla chips and freshly popped popcorn with real butter). Perhaps I would have dropped the weight faster by avoiding these foods; however, I didn't want to feel that I was constantly depriving myself of foods I love. There had to be a balance.

I start my mornings with a tall glass of water with fresh-squeezed lemon (one half lemon) and honey (1/2 teaspoon), for a great liver cleanse. No sooner than 30 minutes later, I have my morning coffee with unsweetened coconut milk. After my morning walk, I enjoy my breakfast smoothie. Late morning, I have my lunch smoothie. Mid-afternoon, I have a high-protein snack (organic celery with hummus and pumpkin seeds or two scrambled eggs with fresh fruit). For dinner, I have either my dinner smoothie or a healthy dinner option (meat with vegetables). The wonderful thing about this approach is that I can do this every day of my life. I also don't feel deprived, and I'm eating healthy food. As of the publishing of this book, I am 6 months into maintenance, and I've been able to be within 2-5 pounds of my lowest weight.

Another food factor came when I took a hair sensitivity test that tested for 975 food and environmental sensitivities. It was recommended to me by Leisa Pimm, and I will be forever grateful. Just mail in a few pieces of your hair, and your results will be emailed to you in a couple of weeks. I learned that I had a sensitivity to dairy, whole wheat flour, mangos, pumpkin, sweet potatoes, gelatin, and basil, to name a few. No wonder my grandmother's pumpkin pie recipe upsets my stomach! It has dairy in the whipped cream topping, whole wheat flour in the crust, and gelatin and pumpkin in the filling! It's super fun going to a restaurant and telling the waiter that I can't have dairy or anything made with whole wheat flour. They look at me as if I have three heads.

Bill was quite skeptical of the hair test. He said the only reason that mangos showed up on my results was because I was eating mangos every day in my smoothies (prior to substituting them for peaches). After his hair test results came back, and rabbit showed up as one of his food sensitivities, I told him that he should stop eating rabbits! (Although plentiful in our neighborhood, Bill doesn't actually eat them.)

Since I took the hair test and removed sensitive foods from my diet, my belly has been much flatter, and I feel better. A few months ago, I had a day when I regressed into anti-healthy eating and ate two mozzarella sticks and a small serving of mac-n-cheese. Within 30 minutes, my belly was bloated, and I had to unbutton my jeans. The reaction was so sudden and obvious that I haven't had much dairy or whole wheat flour since. It's just not worth it. If you'd like to learn about your own food sensitivities, you can purchase the test at allergytest.co (not dot com). As an aside, I have a friend who eats bagels every day of her life, and she doesn't get a bloated belly. Obviously, she doesn't have a sensitivity to wheat. Since ridding my diet of my sensitive foods, it is pretty awesome not to look pregnant, especially since I am over 50!

In the spirit of building a lifestyle that I could do forever, I drank alcohol during my weight loss journey. Depending on the day, I might enjoy a glass of Chardonnay or a Skinny Margarita. Just keeping it real! I've continued this approach in maintenance. I think it's a mistake to completely rid yourself of foods or drinks you love and enjoy if you plan to go back to them after reaching your weight loss goal. I believe it's better to figure out how they play into your new, healthier lifestyle and find the balance now. Otherwise, you'll risk rebounding later.

For the first 12 months, I didn't use any apps to track my calories or exercise. After doing the first few interviews for this book, I realized that apps might be helpful. I began using FitBit to track my exercise and MyFitnessPal to track my calories.

In the past, I hated counting calories. I don't like the micromanaging aspect that calorie trackers represent. However, I wanted to be honest about the exact foods I was putting in my body and how many calories I was consuming. It was a real revelation to see the number of calories in the "healthy" foods I was eating; for instance, I often had ½ a cup of pumpkin seeds and ½ a cup of chopped dates for a snack. I was shocked to realize there are 320 calories in ½ a cup of pumpkin seeds and 520 calories in ½ a cup of chopped dates. I was eating 840 calories in one snack!

FitBit shows me the number of calories I'm burning daily. Depending on my level of exercise, I burn between 2,000–2,500 calories in a day (on average). This information is helpful as I determine the right number of calories to eat daily. I strive to stay between 1,200 and 1,500 calories per day.

When I am faced with attending a party, holiday event, or traveling, I always plan ahead. Planning ahead is the secret to success in these circumstances. For parties, I usually eat before I go so I don't show up starving. If I have no idea what will be served, I will take along a few healthy snacks that I can enjoy during the party. If it's one of my friend's houses, I usually know what they tend to serve, and there are always healthy options available. Recently, I attended a party and brought my own white wine because the hostess prefers red wine. Drinking red wine upsets my stomach due to the high sugar content. A nice Chardonnay is low in sugar and sits well in my system. Of course, I could have decided not to drink at this party, but I wanted the option, so I planned for it.

For traveling, I absolutely bring my own food for the plane and don't rely on the airport having the right types of food. Going through airport security with food in your bag is always fun. Just today, I went through security with my gluten-free pasta and beef marinara sauce. My food was flagged, but as soon as they saw what it was, they let me go. I'll usually make a joke to the TSA security person that getting flagged is the price I pay to eat healthily and that I can't find the same food in the airport. For food during my trip, I plan my menu ahead of time. I'll bring pre-measured bags of pumpkin seeds, dried dates, and gluten-free fruit bars for snacks. I'll buy hard-boiled eggs at a local grocery store and enjoy that for breakfast with instant oatmeal (yes, I know instant oatmeal is processed. I can't usually make my smoothies when traveling unless I'm staying at a house with a blender.) For lunch, I opt for a healthy salad if we're eating out. For dinner, I opt for a meat dish with vegetables. I commit to eating well on my trip and staying away from foods that aren't helpful. When I'm successful with that approach, I feel great, and I return from my travels within 1-2 pounds higher than my pre-trip weight.

For holidays and special events, I'll either help plan the menu and include healthy options, or I'll eat ahead of time and bring my own healthy snacks. Sometimes, I will allow myself to have one or two not-so-healthy options if I really want them. However, I am so sold on my new, smaller self (who doesn't look pregnant) that I don't want to risk it and eat foods that my body doesn't like. I was recently at a wedding where they were serving popcorn coated with Mother's Circus Animal Cookies with the special pink and white icing. Oh my gosh! That was so decadent! I had to try some. I almost put a piece in my mouth that included part of the cookie. As soon as I realized it, I put that piece down and only ate the pieces with popcorn and icing. I didn't want to risk eating anything with whole wheat flour and have my belly bloat. While I avoided any foods that I'm sensitive to, I fully enjoyed the foods I could eat and the white wine that was served with the meal!

I don't have any issues with staying on my weight loss journey during illness. Fortunately, I had only one minor cold, and I was easily able to stay on course with my healthy eating. Again, when you make it your "lifestyle" and not a short-term diet, you just keep doing what you've been doing, and you don't skip a beat. Plus, I find it easier for my body to fight infection if I'm feeding it healthy foods.

Oh, the blessed plateau! Or should that be the cursed plateau? I thought I had hit a plateau when my body would not fall lower than 156 pounds. While my original goal was to hit 150 pounds, I hit a 50-pound weight loss when I hit 156 pounds (if you consider the three extra pounds from my clothes and walking boot that I was wearing for my high weight of 209 pounds). Thinking that I was at a plateau, I called Russ Powell (the Licensed Nutritionist later profiled in this book) and asked her what was going on. She asked me where I had come up with my goal of weighing 150 pounds. I told her it was based on the standard height and weight charts. She immediately exclaimed, "Those numbers are for Chinese people!" Then she calculated my ideal weight based on my age and height. She told me that my ideal weight was between 152-158 pounds, and my ideal daily calorie intake was 1,200-1,800 calories. I really appreciated her expertise and feedback. It is so helpful working with someone who specializes in something I know little about. That's the beauty of a coach! I didn't so much hit a plateau as I had hit a new low to which my body had to adjust. I am incredibly happy at this weight, and if I go lower, great; if I don't, that's fine too. Different people profiled in this book have much to say about plateaus, so keep reading!

Throughout my journey, the way I put myself back on track before I felt like it was "too late" or I had "fallen off the wagon" was simply to have conversations with myself about where I was in my journey and why my weight might have gone up that day or over a few days. If I had two or three days in a row in which my weight went up, I would just consider what had been transpiring in my life. Had I been eating salty foods? Had I been sleeping well? Was I under stress? Had I been traveling? There are so many factors that go into our daily weight that everything must be considered.

After a day of poor eating, I would say to myself, "Tomorrow is a new day, and I will do better." When the weight went up, I would say, "That's okay. You're good." When I was tempted to eat something I shouldn't, I would ask myself, "Is it really worth it?" or I'd simply state, "It's not worth it," or, "I'm good, I don't need it."

Overall, my internal conversation around my weight loss journey has been positive. I never beat myself up emotionally or mentally. I just encourage myself to keep at it and figure out which foods give me the best results. Once I learned about my food sensitivities, I made a commitment to stay away from those foods as much as possible. I gave up mangos in my daily lunch smoothie immediately. I have also learned to live without dairy and whole wheat foods. I have friends and family who took the food sensitivity test and declared that they were not going to stop eating certain foods that showed up in their results by saying, "I like that food too much." I understand having a deep attachment to certain foods – heck, I can't eat cheese anymore unless I want to bloat! But why would you take a test like that, get your results, and then not even try removing sensitive foods from your diet? I get it; it's a process. It takes time to reach your limit when you are willing to do "anything" to get healthy and lose the extra weight. I had to find my limit, and everyone else must do the same.

My friends and family were supportive of my weight loss. I didn't make a big deal about beginning my weight loss journey; I just quietly began by changing the foods I was eating. When they saw my results, their support grew. Most people want to see you successful for a period of time before believing you are committed. Once they know you are in it to win it, their level of support increases.

When I cook for the family, I choose healthy recipes that everyone can enjoy. That being said, my husband, Bill, does most of the cooking. He cooks recipes he and the kids enjoy and also cooks healthy options for me. Not eating dairy and whole wheat flour has been tricky. He will excitedly tell me about a dinner menu he wants to cook, only to have me point out all the dairy and whole wheat flour in those recipes. I just tell him that I'll figure out what I can eat from the menu he has created. I don't think it's fair for me to ask him to change what he wants to cook for the family. I can usually get enough to eat from what he's cooking and what we already have in the house. I never wanted my new lifestyle to create issues for the family. If they want to eat healthier with me, that's great, but I was never going to force it on them. Fortunately, when I do cook, they enjoy my recipes, too.

The one thing I wish I had known at the beginning of my weight loss journey that I know now is, I wish I had known that it was absolutely going to work! I wish I had known that I would successfully lose fifty pounds in one year and get my body back. There were so many unknown facts in the beginning, and I worried about it "turning out like last time" when I lost only 10-15 pounds and then gained it back immediately. The important thing about including success stories from other people who lost 50 pounds after age 50 is that you're not just reading about one person who had success. You will be reading stories of multiple people who did it and how they did it. You will also hear from a Medical Doctor who discusses the problems that excess weight causes and how losing weight positively affects your dependence on prescription medications, a Registered and Licensed Dietician who helps people find success every day by losing weight and drastically reducing their A1C levels, and a previous professional weight loss coach with her own story of successful weight loss.

I've had some fantastic results from my weight loss journey. I no longer deal with asthma. Prior to my weight loss, I had to be on a daily preventative inhaler and use a rescue inhaler when I walked in cold temperatures. My asthma doctor and I agreed for me to stop taking the preventative medication during the summer to see if I needed to use only that inhaler during the colder months. Since losing weight and walking in very cold temperatures (down in the 20s) this past winter, I haven't had any issues with asthma. When I didn't need my daily inhaler or my rescue inhaler at all, I was excited! My lung function is now strong, and I haven't had any flare-ups.

All my cholesterol numbers have improved over the year following my weight loss. You can see from the chart below that my total cholesterol number dropped from 169 in 2022 to 102 in 2023. My triglycerides decreased from 161 to 49 in 2023. My HDL, VLDL and LDL cholesterol numbers all greatly improved over the same time-period. Truly amazing!

	Healthy Range	2022	2023
Total Cholesterol	100-199	169	102
Triglycerides	0-149	161	49
HDL Cholesterol	>39	39	46
VLDL Cholesterol	5-40	28	12
LDL Cholesterol	0-99	102	44

My weight loss hacks:

1. Get your hair tested and stop eating foods that are sensitive to your system.
2. Weigh yourself every day.
3. Claim your new lowest weight.
4. Plan ahead for parties, holidays, and trips.
5. Choose foods you could eat forever.
6. Remove the stress of daily food choices and eat the same foods every day.
7. Take supplements based on the needs of your genes.

One of the things I enjoyed learning about most through the interviews for this book was learning about other people's weight loss hacks. I ended up incorporating many of them, and they really helped me. Instead of naming them here, I will share them at the end of the book. I want you to discover for yourself the things that you feel will be helpful for your own journey.

What's the best part of losing weight? Getting my body back, wearing smaller clothes and looking great! I also love how I feel and the sustained energy levels throughout my day. It is so fun buying super cute clothes in smaller sizes and having them fit well and look good on my new body; I am constantly amazed at how good I look and feel. And yes, it's in that order: #1 Look and #2 Feel. My husband and I recently enjoyed a vacation in Jamaica, and it was so fun wearing bikinis by day and form-fitting dresses by night. I might be 52, but I felt like I was 25! You can't put a price on that! And my health has dramatically improved. Truly a win-win!

Have you heard enough to make a decision? Make the decision, create your plan, and get your body back!

For additional resources, please visit Losing50After50.com.

In the next chapter, you'll hear from Dr. Jeffrey Schaffer, M.D. who shares the effects that excess weight has on all the body systems.

CHAPTER 2
JEFFREY SCHAFFER, M.D.

Dr. Jeffrey Schaffer is one of the "regulars" that I visit in the morning when I walk to Einstein's Bagels. His friends call him "Doc". He is happy to give medical advice to anyone who asks, though he is most gratified when they follow his sage wisdom and achieve good results. He has been an Emergency Room physician since 1988, including 28 years in a Level 1 Trauma unit. He now works part-time in free-standing emergency departments. Doc has been included in this book for his perspective on weight loss as a medical doctor, not as a weight loss success story.

Excess weight affects our health by putting stress on all the systems in the body, including the cardiac/cardiovascular and metabolic (responsible for glucose and fat metabolism) systems. Secondarily, excess weight can lead to diabetes (sustained high blood sugar levels), hypertension (high blood pressure) and high cholesterol/triglycerides, which leads to deterioration in the body's systems. Excessive weight also puts pressure on the joints and back, which can lead to problems later in life, like degenerative joint disease (osteoarthritis) and joint replacement surgeries.

Most people do not want to hear (directly) that they need to lose weight, even from a doctor. They view the information as a criticism. So, Doc takes an indirect approach. When patients have diabetes and hypertension, he will point out that their numbers will improve if they lose weight. While calories in versus calories out is still a good approach to weight loss, nutrition (eating high-quality calories) plays a significant role. Doc feels that nutrition is about 80% of the battle and exercise is 20%.

The body initially burns glucose for fuel and then burns fat. All successful diets come down to getting past the glucose metabolism pathway and into the fat metabolism pathway as quickly as possible. You must choose the right foods in the right ratios and let your body do the rest. Doc believes it's important to keep the body in ketosis, and a ketone breath meter can be helpful to track ketones. A ketone breath meter can be purchased on Amazon. He shared that you want to stay away from the extreme and malignant stage of ketosis known as ketoacidosis. Another name for this is known as diabetic ketoacidosis, which is due to a lack of insulin resulting in excessive ketones in the body. As a good rule, always seek advice from a medical professional when attempting a weight loss journey.

In order to lose weight, one needs to eat less, eat the right combination of foods (no bread or sugars), and eat foods higher in protein. However, he made the point that eating fat is usually not the issue in gaining weight. When you eat foods high in fat, the fat is metabolized and turned into glucose, then stored as glycogen. The body burns glycogen, and the excess glycogen is then put into fat storage. A diet low in carbs and high in protein is helpful. The body uses more energy to break down proteins than carbs.

Though he doesn't tell people to use any particular apps, like FitBit, food diaries can be useful when tracking weight loss. He feels that weight loss apps can be helpful for people who want to be diligent about what they are eating.

In terms of plateaus, it is normal for you to lose more weight in the beginning and for weight loss to level off later. You cannot eat microscopic amounts of food forever; you must find a balance of foods you like to eat for the long haul. Walking 30 minutes per day is helpful. Another way to beat the plateau is to add resistance training to your weekly workouts. Resistance training will build muscle, which increases your basal metabolic rate (BMR), which is the number of calories your body burns to keep all systems functioning. Being "skin and bones" will lower your BMR. Building muscle will increase your BMR, and lean muscle burns more calories as you sleep! You can measure your BMR with a RENPHO Smart Scale. It measures weight, BMI, body fat, subcutaneous fat, visceral fat, body water, skeletal muscle, muscle mass, bone mass, protein, BMR, metabolic age, and fat-free body weight. The scale sends all the data to an app on your phone that tracks everything for you. You can find this specialized scale on Amazon for about $20.00. Not bad!

Overweight people in their 50s, 60s, and 70s are often on multiple medications. They take oral hypoglycemic drugs for non-insulin-dependent diabetes (like Metformin), hypertension prescriptions (like Lisinopril), and statin medication for cholesterol issues (like Atorvastatin). Doc clarifies that being under a doctor's supervision does not mean that the doctor is telling you how to lose weight; it means that they are monitoring your body and how prescribed medications are reacting to your new lower weight. For instance, they will monitor your blood pressure, and if it is too low, they might change the dosage of your medication. He noted that overall cholesterol levels might not come down since it is a function of lower weight and genetics. Triglycerides should decrease when you lose weight (mine dropped from 161 to 49 in twelve months).

Doc's weight loss hacks:

1. If you are following a weight loss system, modify it to your personal food preferences that fit the program.

2. Use a ketone breath meter to ensure that you are in a healthy stage of ketosis.

3. Use a smart scale (like the RENPHO Smart Scale) to track your progress.

4. Find healthy foods you can eat at restaurants (like grilled chicken and green beans).

5. Cook three eggs a day in healthy oils, specifically organic MCT C8 oil and avocado oil, with a higher burning point.

6. Do not eat the chips at Mexican restaurants. Eat the fajita meat with grilled vegetables as an easy alternative.

7. Do not try to lose weight alone. Find other people you can do it with or get an accountability partner, as this makes the journey easier.

Are you ready to choose in favor of your health? Make the decision, create your plan, and get your body back!

For additional resources, please visit Losing50After50.com.

In the next chapter, you'll hear from Russ, who helps her clients win the weight and diabetes management battle every day.

CHAPTER 3
RUSS POWELL – REGISTERED & LICENSED DIETICIAN

R uss and I met through a professional business networking group. I immediately liked her and her great energy. We became instant friends after sharing lunch and learning about each other's backgrounds. Russ is a Registered and Licensed Dietician who specializes in weight management and diabetes. She is a Certified Diabetes Care Education Specialist. Russ has been helping people win the weight and diabetes management battle for the past 13 years. She is included in this book as a professional who helps people manage their weight and diabetes, not as a weight loss success story.

Excess weight can have a significant impact on chronic illnesses like diabetes. Russ shared that 1 in 3 people have prediabetes and 1 in 10 people, who are 20 years or older, have diabetes. These numbers are projected to increase by 700% over the next 40 years. Sadly, the diabetes diagnosis is hitting people at much earlier ages than in the past and is projected to continue in the coming decades.

Russ began her career in a corporate hospital setting. Her clients were struggling with diabetes on a regular basis. She realized that doctors were giving them a restrictive food list and a prescription for medication. These people were coming back week after week and were not getting better. She wanted to help them, so she would spend an extra 10 minutes with her clients and educate them on healthy food choices and what they needed to do to win the diabetic game. Soon thereafter, her clients weren't coming back for more medication because they were getting healthy!

It was frustrating for Russ to only spend about 10-15 minutes with each of her hospital clients. Furthermore, she was seeing around 20 people per day. She didn't feel the environment was very patient-centered. So, Russ began her own private practice. She spends an adequate amount of time with her clients now and truly works to understand how they got to where they are. Initially, she had to run through a checklist for doctors; now, she calls her work "intensive," where she truly gets to know her clients and helps them on an individual basis. She helps them move from a victim mindset to a solution mindset. Together, they create a roadmap to get them to a much better place for their health.

Russ has three types of clients: 1) those who are pre-diabetic; 2) others who have had Type 2 diabetes for years; and 3) clients with what she calls "denial-betes" (they have diabetes but have denied it, never made a change to their diet and now they feel worse than they've ever felt). Her claim to fame is that she has helped her clients put Type 2 Diabetes into remission. Wow!

When asked about the percentage of nutrition to exercise, in terms of the effect on weight loss, she said 75-80% of weight loss is affected by nutrition. Hands down. It is hard to outwork a bad diet. It's not just about calories in versus calories out. It also depends on the stage of life one is in. For exercise, there are differences between fat loss and weight loss. To burn calories, cardio is best. To maintain weight loss, you need 2-3 days per week of resistance training. Russ likens cardio to a debit card swipe and resistance training to investing in a 401K. When you burn calories through cardio, it helps to create a calorie deficit for the day. When you burn calories through resistance training, you continue burning calories, even after your workout! She encourages 3-4 days of cardio and 2-3 days of resistance training each week.

Russ says to celebrate plateaus! Plateaus are very normal and often happen every 20-30 pounds lost. It's important to learn your body's rhythm and not freak out when you hit a plateau. A plateau represents your body settling into your new, lower weight. You've done enough consistent work to reach this milestone, and your body has to catch up! She tells her clients not to worry about a 1–2-week plateau. When a plateau continues for four weeks or longer, she counsels her clients to move away from the scale in terms of making their weight the only focal point for success. Are your pants getting looser? Is your bra falling off? Is your waist getting smaller? Are your shoes feeling bigger? (Who knew?! Your feet can lose weight too!) However, if you're not seeing any of these other signs, it's time to reassess and change things up. Are you doing the same type of exercise? Are you eating the same foods? Our bodies can get stuck when there is little variety, so go shift a few things!

In terms of moving away from the scale, Russ said that it's important to have a good relationship with the scale. You cannot let the number on the scale determine your value. Focus on everything good that is happening with your weight loss: better energy, looser clothes, hitting lower weight milestones, etc. Mindset is critical. You've got to stay positive and say nice things to yourself. If there are negative voices in your head, counseling can be extremely helpful.

In maintenance, you must have a plan for after you hit the number! So often, people are solely focused on a number (their weight loss goal) but have no plan for after they accomplish their goal.

Russ doesn't recommend any weight loss programs, per se. She is not in favor of rule-based programs which say, "Eat this, don't eat that," or programs based on points. She believes these programs cause people to become disconnected from themselves and can lead to disordered eating patterns. For example, if you're full at 7:00 p.m. but you have a snack scheduled at 8:00 p.m., don't eat the snack! It's so important to learn to be connected to your body. Some days you might need less food, and other days you might need a little more food. If you're so focused on the rules and not on what your body needs, you're going to have a tough time.

Russ helps her clients create a custom lifestyle plan, not a "diet." Proteins, whole-grain carbohydrates, and healthy fats are the components of a successful plan. For clients with more weight to lose, she recommends a diet high in plant-based foods. Plants fill up the gaps in your stomach, make you fuller and help you return to fat burning more quickly. She calls this a plant-forward approach. While not every meal is plant-based, she helps clients add more plant meals to their weekly schedule. Interestingly, my smoothie recipes are 100% plant-based, and I've had significant success with this approach to eating.

There are no specific foods that Russ tells her clients to stay away from. She doesn't use the word "can't" because then that's all you'll focus on. Overall, she encourages people to monitor their intake of high-sodium foods (deli meats, soups, bread, crackers, pizza, hamburgers, etc.). Foods high in sodium can make your brain think you are hungry when you aren't. People who are sensitive to salt can put on 2-3 pounds a day when their diet is high in sodium, and the weight will persist! She counsels her clients to limit the intake of meat that comes from four-legged animals (no, not your cat or dog) and things that have a heartbeat. Meat that comes from four-legged animals often causes an inflammatory response. Instead, eat chicken, fish, and plants.

Russ is a fan of tracking apps, such as Fitbit, Apple Health, MyFitnessPal, LoseIt!, and My Food Diary, plus she sees them as excellent accountability tools. People often overestimate how much they move and underestimate how much they eat. As long as you are using the data as data, these apps can be helpful. As soon as you tie any personal value to your results, these apps can become detrimental to your mindset and well-being. Instead, use the apps as an awareness tool and use the data to make informed decisions on your plan.

I downloaded Fitbit and MyFitnessPal after 12 months. Tracking the calories expended through exercise and the caloric intake from food was a game changer! I was shocked at how many calories were in the foods I was eating. While I was eating pretty clean, I would snack on different foods, and some of those foods were high in calories, for example, tortilla chips. I love tortilla chips, but 5.5 Tostitos Chips are 70 calories. I'm not sure I have ever eaten just 5.5 tortilla chips in one sitting. My average is closer to 22 chips (minimum), which is 280 calories! Even healthy snacks like pumpkin seeds and dates are high in calories. Pumpkin seeds are 160 calories for a ¼ cup serving and dates are 130 calories for a 1.5 ounce serving (equal to 1/8 cup). Prior to tracking my calories, I was eating closer to a ½ cup serving of each. Once I began journalling my food intake, my food choices changed, and I immediately began losing weight again after a plateau. My personal approach to journalling is that if you're willing to eat it, you should be willing to track it in your food journal. If you're not willing to track it, don't put it in your mouth!

Russ has a database with thousands of recipes that she tailors to her clients' needs. She has recipes for busy, on-the-go clients. She has menu recommendations for other clients who eat out often. Her favorite recipe websites are SkinnyTaste. com, AllRecipes.com, and Eatingwell.com. A few years ago, I purchased the book: *Simple Green Meals: 100+ Plant-Powered Recipes to Thrive from the Inside Out* by Jen Hansard. It has healthy recipes and options for transforming them into gluten-free, dairy-free, and vegan meals.

When her clients hit their goal weight and enter maintenance, Russ encourages them to focus on staying within a 5-pound maintenance range. Plan for your weight to fluctuate within that range. If you go above the top number, then it's time to look at what you are eating and make necessary changes. Know that it takes your body one year to fully reset to your new lower weight. Also, it's important to eat different foods and keep the variety. It's essential to keep exercising and do resistance training. Russ says to do "spot checks" on your eating and exercising once a quarter by tracking your food and exercise for one week. Have you become lax and are you snacking more? It's good to review what you've been doing and keep yourself on track. She likens the "spot check" to a quarterly business review. Treat your health like your business.

If you go out of your range, don't freak out! Do a balance assessment. How are you prioritizing work? Are you in a social season? Has your sleep been off? Are you working out regularly? Have you been going out to eat more than you cook at home? Take three days to reflect. She calls this a 3-day relapse prevention plan. Weight usually creeps up when you've lost your balance. It's easy to be so excited about your new smaller size that you want to celebrate and maybe you overdo it. You've got to get back to a lifestyle that is sustainable and allows you to stay in your target weight range.

Holidays can be rough! Decide ahead of time: Are you taking time off your eating regimen? What part of your new lifestyle can you continue through this time? Can you bring a healthy dish to the gathering? Can you pack food for a trip? Can you eat at the same time? Pick and choose things that you have control over and give yourself compassion and grace.

It's also important to be armored with comebacks when your friends and family make their comments about your new smaller size. What are you going to say when they comment on your food choices? Like, if you want to eat a piece of pie, they might say, "I thought you were dieting. Why are you eating a piece of pie?" Know that the comments will come, so be ready for them. It will take time for your family and friends to adjust to your new life.

Cooking for your family, but you want to stay on your plan? Russ suggests you make a menu for the week and ask for feedback. Do not be a short-order cook. Set the expectation that you're happy to cook the food they like; you'll just need their help with the food preparation. Get your kids involved and teach them how to cook! They'll need this important skill in college and later in life. Russ eats a plant-based diet, and her husband likes meat. So, she will cook the vegetables, and he will cook the meat. She likes to batch cook on Sunday (for the week), and her husband will cook a "Dad meal" during the week for himself and their son. She also asks them to find recipes they like from her database so that she can cook for the family. Bottomline, have a plan, get everyone involved, and set healthy boundaries!

At the beginning of a weight loss journey, remember it's a marathon, not a sprint. You might want to lose a certain amount of weight in a specific time, but life goes on. It's good to assess how you've done with diets in the past. When did you fail? What worked? What didn't work? Why are you doing this now? Decide how it's going to be different this time. Russ has her clients write a contract letter to themselves. When things aren't going well, she has them review their contract to keep them on track.

She also collaborates with her clients on barrier busters. #1 Barrier Buster: I overeat when I'm distracted. So, instead of sitting down to watch TV with a whole bag of chips, you sit down with a pre-portioned bowl of chips. Or you choose not to watch TV while eating any food. #2 Barrier Buster: When work gets tough, I stop exercising. Plan your exercise at the beginning of your day and begin work afterward. Or schedule your exercise as an appointment on your calendar and treat it as a non-negotiable. Be proactive!

When your weight loss journey is lifestyle-driven and health-focused, your medications will often change – for the better! When you lose weight, you'll have a dosage reduction because dosages are often based on your weight. Also, you will likely reduce the total amount of medications that you take regularly. Be sure to seek guidance from your healthcare professional before making any changes to your medications. As a rule, it's a good idea to check in with your prescribing physician at least once every 3-4 months during your weight loss journey.

If you don't make time for your health, you'll be forced to take time for your disease. If your exercise appointment was an appointment for dialysis to keep you alive, would you skip it? An average dialysis appointment lasts 4-5 hours per day, 5-7 days per week. Would you rather sign up for that or sign up for 30 minutes of daily exercise that could keep you from having to do dialysis? Instead of only looking at today, it is critical you consider what today's choices could bring in the future – good or bad.

Russ is a huge supporter of systems and rewards. You've got to put systems in place that will fuel you. For example, I walk 5 miles almost every day. I am out the door by 6:00 a.m. with my coconut milk in a small container and an empty coffee tumbler. I walk 2 miles to my local Einstein's Bagels. I buy a coffee refill (for half the price of a regular coffee) and add my coconut milk. I visit with the regular customers who are there each morning. I don't eat bagels due to my wheat flour sensitivity. After engaging with them for 15-20 minutes, I walk home for 2 miles and then walk a "final mile" in the neighborhood. I feel fantastic after my walk, with my exercise done for the day, usually by 7:45 a.m. My system is walking, and my reward is coffee and enjoyable conversation.

Russ's weight loss hacks:

1. If you're hungry and it's been less than 3 hours, ask yourself if it's head hunger or physical hunger. Head hunger is extremely specific. For example, you want something salty, sweet, crunchy, or fatty. Physical hunger is not as specific. Your stomach might be growling, you feel weak, and you've already had plenty of water. It's probably time to eat. On average, she suggests eating every 4 hours. If you have physical hunger before 4 hours is up, you probably didn't eat enough at your last meal, so go ahead and eat something. Tip: if it's head hunger, find a 20-minute distraction and change the scene.

2. Strategize your barrier busters.

Final thoughts...do what is right for you. Don't necessarily do exactly what someone else has done. It's also important to be around like-minded people. Have a good support system. Find people who you can bounce ideas and gain perspective from. Remember, this is a marathon, not a sprint. Setbacks are not bad; they can help you learn and grow.

Do you want to connect with Russ?
Find her online at RussPowellNutrition.com.
Her Instagram is @fatlossdiabetesdietician.

Are you hoping to avoid diabetes? Make the decision, create your plan, and get your body back!

For additional resources, please visit Losing50After50.com.

In the next chapter, you'll hear from Candi, who literally had to drink lidocaine every day in order to manage the pain from her leaky gut syndrome prior to losing 65 pounds.

CHAPTER 4
CANDI'S STORY

C andi and I have known each other for many years. Our boys were in Boy Scouts together. She was one of my inspirations when I saw her losing weight and getting her body back.

Candi began her most recent weight loss journey at age 52. She is 5'7" and weighed 290 pounds when she began. Over the past three years, she has lost 65 pounds. She would like to lose another 40 to 60 more pounds, but she's not focused on a specific number. Her "ideal" weight, according to doctors, is between 135-150 pounds. However, her German genetics are not going to let that happen. The last time she weighed within that range, she was 14 years old and starving herself at 1,000 calories per day.

Candi had dieted in the past. She would go up 50 pounds and then lose 30 pounds. After marriage, she gained weight with each pregnancy and could not lose it all. Candi got more serious about her weight after passing the 50-year mark. She was more focused on the endgame. She wanted to be there for her grandchildren and be able to play with them on the floor. Before age 50, she wasn't thinking about these types of things.

In her late 40s, Candi had Leaky Gut Syndrome, was depressed, and felt physically bad overall. Her gut hurt so much that she was drinking Lidocaine every day to reduce the pain. She was in poor health, and her body was shutting down. She was on a drug that blocked the acid production in her stomach, another drug that blocked the hormone that triggered her stomach to produce acid, an elixir that would coat her stomach from the acid not being produced (to prevent ulcers), and she was drinking lidocaine (called "magic") that was ordinarily used to numb your skin for stitches or a shot.

Though Candi didn't follow a specific program, she joined a gym and met with a nutritionist. To find out what she could do to heal herself, she took a blood test to determine food sensitivities. She learned that she was sensitive to 23 foods, including gluten and dairy. She shared that when you are eating foods that your system is sensitive to, it's like giving your body a thousand paper cuts. One paper cut is fine, but a thousand can wreak havoc and cause inflammation. Her nutritionist asked her to give up the sensitive foods for 12 weeks. Candi did it, and at the 12-week mark (also 4th of July), she ate a cheeseburger on a gluten-free bun and instantly regretted it. She felt bad for three days. She then made the decision to go one year without eating any of the sensitive foods on her list. She didn't lose a lot of weight but was taken off the majority of her regular prescription medications and felt much better.

She also studied the Noom program and learned the psychology behind why you eat. She was inspired to create her ultimate "why", which is about creating the life you want to live. She wanted to be able to go anywhere and do anything. Candi loves nature walks, rollercoaster rides, and wants to be able to get on the ground with her future grandchildren and play with them without being in pain. Once she focused on her physical health and how she felt, she was able to lose weight.

At age 52, Candi lost 20 pounds, but she wanted to lose more. At age 53, she had a friend, who is a Kinesiologist, who asked her to get serious about losing the extra weight. At that point, she had been eating better and exercising. Her friend said that wasn't enough and she needed to reset her metabolism. He suggested she do intermittent fasting and skip breakfast each day. He explained that the body wasn't designed to eat every 4 hours, around the clock. She began intermittent fasting and made a goal to do it for 28 straight days.

Her friend also introduced her to Mark Sisson of MarksDailyApple.com. She credits Mark Sisson for teaching her the functions of the body and how to do intermittent fasting effectively. On his website, Mark has an introduction to the intermittent fasting program with a 28-day structure. Through her friend and Mark, Candi was given an extraordinary education on how the body works and why certain approaches to weight loss work better than others. Candi also mentioned a great podcast that Mark Sisson did with Joe Rogan. I Googled "Joe Rogan Mark Sisson podcast" and found multiple podcasts they've done. You can do the same; search and listen to their conversations. After Candi committed to the intermittent fasting lifestyle, she dropped 50 pounds in one year.

For her intermittent fasting plan, Candi doesn't eat breakfast. Her first meal is sometime between 12:00 p.m.-2:00 p.m., and she has a salad with protein. Between 4:30 p.m.-6:00 p.m., she will have a snack to hold her over until dinner at 7:30 p.m. For snacks, she loves almond crackers with protein like goat cheese or beef jerky.

Candi doesn't eat gluten, dairy, or sugar. She uses stevia in her coffee and monk fruit in place of sugar in recipes. She also eliminated coconut, cauliflower, and corn (for the most part). She will eat corn on an extremely limited basis since it is known to cause inflammation in the body. She'll eat the occasional white potato.

Candi only eats organic, non-GMO food, wild-caught fish, and naturally raised meat. She eats all kinds of meat, including steak and fish. She shared that she eats the whole gamut of protein and includes protein at every meal. She also enjoys foods from Mark Sisson's "Primal Kitchen". Candi uses higher-quality oils for cooking, like avocado or Italian olive oils. It matters which fats you put in your body. She is happier to spend the additional money now (on healthy food) than spend money on medical expenses, prescriptions, and doctors in the future. Candi agrees, *"If you don't pay for your health now, you'll pay for your disease later."*

Candi enjoys good wine, so she did not eliminate wine from her diet. She also loves margaritas and would make her own with tequila, fresh lime juice, and stevia. Another favorite of hers is vodka, fresh lemon juice, and soda water. Candi bought a SodaStream for her home and loves making flavored water. Water with fresh-squeezed lemon is one of her go-to daily drinks. She also loves whiskey and bourbon, which she enjoys in moderation.

For exercise, Candi walks on the treadmill four times per week for 30 to 45 minutes. Her goal is to do "regular movement". She also loves weightlifting and feels it was and is pivotal to her weight loss success. She can hike 5 miles and out-walk anyone with speed. She can also carry a case of whiskey with no problem!

To stay successful through the holidays, Candi would do her best to stay within the parameters of her base diet. She would have no gluten or dairy. She would also be the one to cook so that she would have something healthy to eat.

When eating out at restaurants, she would bring the list of foods she could eat and ask the chef to recommend a dish for her. Many restaurants were happy to accommodate. Since it's difficult to control the quality of food at restaurants, she wouldn't eat out much.

When working through a plateau, she would focus on her "why" and remember how much she wants to play with her future grandchildren, hiking in Yosemite, walking along the beach (and not falling over), and not having to rely on someone else to do things for her that she should be able to do herself. She learned that our bodies have weight memory, and our weight loss will settle at a previous weight. Our weight will go up one pound, down two pounds, up three pounds, down one pound, etc. From Mark Sisson, she learned that she had to stress her body to break out of a plateau. She found success by shaking things up. She ate different foods, changed the hours of her intermittent fasting, and changed the structure of when she ate different foods (i.e., the time of day when she ate fats, proteins, or carbs). Force your body to learn a new routine, and you will break through the plateau.

Candi's immediate family was supportive of her wanting to be healthier. They did not want her to be sick. Her parents were less supportive and wanted her to make the family recipes the same way they've always been made. Everyone learned to adjust. Her immediate family chose to go to their favorite restaurants when she travelled. Candi would modify recipes to fit what she could eat. They struck a balance with Candi cooking recipes the family loved, but she wouldn't eat the food she made. She also made recipes everyone would eat.

She stressed that this is not a "diet" or a "weight loss program". Her healthier approach to food had to be a lifestyle change. It wasn't helpful to "cheat" on her new lifestyle because it caused her to feel bloated and retain water. Whenever she chose poor eating, she paid for it for days or weeks. When you can correlate food choices to feeling ill, it's much easier to rid your diet of those foods. I shared earlier that my grandmother's pumpkin chiffon pie recipe includes four foods that I have a sensitivity to: pumpkin, wheat flour, dairy, and gelatin. No wonder I felt sick to my stomach when I ate that pie! I didn't feel sick when I was younger, but as I grew older, my sensitivities strengthened. Candi shared that, as we age, it's harder and harder for our bodies to deal with our food sensitivities. It's just not worth it to not eat well.

Candi is saddened for people who choose to eat foods that aren't good for them. They know these foods are bad for them, but they choose to eat them anyway. She knows that they are poisoning themselves with their poor food choices. She has a family member who is in the hospital every three months. They know what they should do to adjust their diet for the better, but they refuse to do it.

Candi wished she had known early on that she was going to feel so good. She also wished she had known the true benefits of exercise in general and weightlifting in particular. She loves the endorphins she gets from a good workout. She genuinely believes her weight loss journey is a lifestyle and not a short-term diet.

Candi had medication changes because of her weight loss, healthy eating, and omitting sensitive foods from her diet. She was able to get off those four drugs and is currently on the lowest dose of her blood pressure medication. She also has one prescription so that she can eat tomatoes (which she will eat once a month). Candi's fasting glucose level dropped from 106 to 93 mg/dL, and her A1C decreased from 5.8% to 5.5%.

She is positive with her internal conversation. She tells herself, "Look how far you've come. I can do this. I've proven to myself that I can do this. I've been doing this for three years." If she knows she's going on a trip with the girls, she'll give herself the license to not eat perfectly. She enjoys herself and then detoxes after the trip and gets back to the healthy pattern afterward. She no longer chastises herself, thanks to years of therapy. During our interview, Candi spoke about her ah-ha moments in counseling and how helpful it was to understand where her thought patterns originated from and whose voice she was listening to (spoiler alert: her mother). She shared that her body is her vehicle in this life, it's how she exists in this dimension, and it's the only one she gets! She realized that she could do anything she wanted to do, and she had to choose what to want. Life doesn't happen to you. You always have choices.

After a day of poor eating, she says to herself, "Okay, that was today, tomorrow is different." When her weight went up, she would say, "Holy shit! Look at that number!" If the higher weight was due to a recent trip, she would be grateful that she had such a wonderful time. Then she would choose to adjust her eating for the day and skip dinner, even if it meant canceling a dinner date. It's not helpful to get down on yourself. It's helpful to find gratitude and focus on the wonderful memories created by the fun trip or experience.

When she is tempted, she would say, "I'm not going to sabotage what I'm doing because of one meal. Congratulations, you respected your body today. You did the right thing for the life you want to live." With foods that make her sick, she would also think, that might look good, but I'll pay for it later.

Candi's weight loss hacks:

1. Eat monk fruit, not processed sugar.

2. Your mouth only tastes the first 3-5 bites of food, after that, the food tastes bland. Only eat food if you can taste it. Stop eating it when you cannot taste it anymore, thereby limiting your caloric intake.

3. Put salad dressing on the fork for each bite, then lettuce. Don't pour salad dressing over the whole salad.

4. Eat a salad every day for lunch. Wash, spin, and chop it ahead of time. Keep it fresh for the week.

5. Have a food plan. Make the plan ahead of time.

6. Habitually use a shopping list. Buy lettuce, mushrooms, peppers, mini cucumbers, and other fresh vegetables.

7. Eat vegetables at every meal.

8. Do intermittent fasting.

9. Don't drink protein shakes high in calories. If protein shakes don't make you feel full, don't drink them. Learn what works best for your body.

10. Avocado oil and Italian olive oils are the best. It matters which oils you put in your body.

What's her favorite part about losing weight? Feeling good in her own skin. She's on her fourth round of new clothes. She also bought a little black dress (for the first time), and it has a belt that draws attention to her waist. She wore that dress with a brand-new pair of boots (the first she purchased in 25 years). She loves it when people say she looks really good. It is just so amazing to feel good in her own skin!

Her concluding thoughts around weight loss are to find gratitude in every situation. Candi really appreciated the support and encouragement she received from advocates and coaches. She felt like she couldn't do it without them. You only get one life! Choose to live!

Are you ready to choose life? Make the decision, create your plan, and get your body back!

For additional resources, please visit Losing50After50.com.

In the next chapter, you'll hear from James, whose highest weight was 568 pounds, and he figured out how to lose 384 of it!

CHAPTER 5
JAMES' STORY

James was referred to me by a mutual friend. She saw my Facebook posts about my desire to interview people who had lost 50 or more pounds after age 50. She suggested I reach out to James. We had a great conversation about his weight loss journey!

James is 5'10" and weighed 568 pounds at age 47. He lost 384 pounds over the course of 4 ½ years. His lowest weight was 184 pounds, but he felt like he looked sick at that weight, so he purposefully gained some weight back. Now, at age 62, he is 210 pounds, though he said his sweet spot is between 190-200 pounds.

James shared that his weight increased from the stress of growing his company from 7 employees to over 200. Along with a lifetime of poor eating habits, he used food as a coping mechanism. He regularly drank 16-25 sodas a day. He would distance himself from things that would make him feel bad or embarrassed. He was very self-conscious and put up a guard. For instance, he was embarrassed when he went to the movie theater, and he couldn't fly on planes because he couldn't fit in the seat, even with seatbelt extenders. A business associate once made a comment to a banker about James that "He's not as dumb as he looks." James felt that people did not see him for him; instead, they only saw the big fat guy. Specifically, he felt his weight held him back in business because potential clients would see him and think, "He can't even take care of himself, much less do anything for us." He was very self-conscious of his weight, and it controlled his life. For work meetings at restaurants, he would arrive early so that he could choose a table with the largest seat instead of being seated in a booth and not being able to fit in it. After years of being heavy, one morning, while standing in front of the mirror, James decided he was tired of being "the fat guy," and it was time for a change.

James did not undergo surgery or use a specific program or any apps to lose weight. He created his own hybrid approach. He read his wife's old Weight Watchers book and learned how to count calories and points. His initial approach was to take in less calories than he burned and exercise regularly. His exercise began with walking to the end of his short driveway and back because that was all he could physically do. Each day he would walk 5-10 more steps than the day before. As he started losing weight, his pace increased. Next, he began running and worked up to a 5K, then a 10K. Then he began biking with a pack of people. This worked well for the first 100-150 pounds. For the next 200 pounds, he hired a personal trainer and added weight training and building muscle. Building muscles burn fat. He worked out three times a day. He loved working out so much that he bought the gym where the trainer worked! He contends that it's a simple formula: you burn more calories than you consume. If you aren't losing weight that way, then you haven't been doing it long enough.

If you've never exercised before, James says to take it slowly, "it's a marathon and not a sprint." The whole weight loss journey is also a marathon. Consider how long it took you to get overweight and to the point where you are; the weight isn't going to come off overnight. "It's like eating a dinosaur, one bite at a time." He suggests walking and listening to music as the best ways to begin exercising.

James avoids soft drinks, cheese, hamburgers with bread, and fries. He also eliminated desserts, sugars, cake, ice cream, starch, and bread. If he is absolutely craving something sweet, he allows himself to eat one Weight Watchers ice cream sandwich.

He eats all types of meats, including chicken, turkey, turkey bacon, and lean beef. He used to drink unsweetened tea, but the caffeine gave him kidney stones, so he stopped drinking caffeinated drinks altogether.

James shared that he and his wife do not eat at home. They always eat out at restaurants. During his weight loss journey, he did not eat anything before lunch. His daily lunch was a 6" turkey sub (from Subway) and water, with a calorie goal of 400-500 calories. For dinner, would eat a chicken breast and green beans, with a calorie goal of 400-500 calories. His daily calorie goal was around 900 calories. He did not drink alcohol during his weight loss journey or during maintenance. He said alcohol is "a glass of calories."

Though they did not usually cook at home, James and his wife loved creating a big spread of food during the holidays. He shared that he dreaded the holidays. His trainer told him to take one day and enjoy the food. On the rare occasion when they would cook at home, James made sure to make food he could eat and served himself smaller portions. He also made sure to avoid food with extra calories, like cheese.

At the higher weight, James slept horribly. He shared that he woke up constantly because he could not breathe and he snored. His sleeping got better as the weight came off. James said he no longer snores at all. He was also sick less frequently. Even colds were brief and minor. After losing weight, James went from multiple regular prescription medications to none. His biggest issue during weight loss was kidney stones. He experienced nine kidney stone episodes. Once he eliminated caffeine, his body stopped producing kidney stones.

James experienced frequent plateaus. He remembered a long plateau when he hit 240 pounds. His trainer told him that it was normal since the body was trying to catch up. Your body must adjust to the new lower weight. Just like a computer stores files, your body stores information on your weight, and it must get rid of the old files. He had to change how he felt about food. Food is for energy and not for pleasure. During his weight loss journey, he weighed himself daily. At first, the weight just melted off, so the daily weigh-in was motivational. After losing some weight, he weighed himself every couple of weeks.

Initially, his family and friends were not very supportive. They would say, "He's on another diet!" They didn't think his new approach would work. But when he was having sustained weight loss, they came around. Both his son and daughter were inspired to lose their extra weight. His wife was supportive and would agree to skip events when James felt that it would not be good to attend. He said it took about two years, but eventually, everyone came around when they realized he was committed to his new healthier lifestyle.

He shared that it was easy to fall off the wagon, especially when attending events that did not serve any healthy foods. He would tell himself to just "get back on the bike" the very next day and not use that event as an excuse. He would remind himself that "It is a lifestyle change."

After a day of poor eating, he would think, "Wow, I can't believe I did that. Tomorrow morning is a new morning." Since he eliminated bad foods from his diet, he rarely had a day of poor eating. When his weight would go up, he would say, "You might have extra water weight," as sore muscles hold onto more water. When he was tempted, he would think, "You got this. Look how far you've come. Focus on walking back into your high school reunion and being the smallest guy." He would also put on headphones and begin power walking anytime he had hunger cravings. He shared that hunger cravings are purely mental. James would also tell himself, "You cannot break. Do not break. You don't need it. What are you going to get from that?"

James' internal conversation around his weight loss journey included focusing on conversations with people who gave him accolades about his lower weight. He did not want to lose his investment. He also kept pictures of guys he wanted to look like. He would tell himself, "Don't mess this up!"

When asked if there was anything he learned late in his weight loss journey that he wished he had known early on, he shared that he wished he had known about the skin surgeries he would have to endure after he lost weight. He wished he had been able to mentally prepare. He had 30 pounds of excess skin, and it took three surgeries to remove it all.

The first surgery was on his upper body. It took 10 hours, and he had nine drains inserted into his body. About ten days later, he waltzed back into the doctor's office (instead of barely being able to walk in and asking for more pain meds) because he was in such good shape from his years of working out. His doctor was in shock at how good he looked and felt. After that, his doctor changed his rules for surgical patients and began requiring them to work out for six weeks prior to surgery.

The second surgery was on his lower body, and it took another 10 hours. The third surgery was for an infected leg, and it took 6 hours. Incredibly, James' pant size decreased from 62 to 31. Now he wears pants that are around 33-34. James felt the surgeries were necessary, even though they were optional. He was quite active, and the extra skin just got in the way. He felt that removing the extra skin aided him in not gaining back all the weight.

Conversely, James shared about a guy he knows who lost hundreds of pounds and was able to compete in Ironman events. He chose not to have the extra skin surgically removed and ended up gaining all the weight back. He now weighs 400 pounds. His friend also drank a considerable amount of alcohol, and James felt that led to the weight coming back.

During maintenance, James sometimes eats turkey bacon for breakfast, a Subway sandwich or chicken wrap for lunch (400-500 calories), and chicken breast and green beans for dinner (700-800 calories). He still works out regularly and weighs himself every couple of weeks. James shared, "My life was built around food. Now it's built around something else."

James' weight loss hacks:

1. Fill a large Yeti with water and add a small amount (1/4 cup) of pre-made Minute Maid lemonade at the beginning of each day (purchase 2-liter bottles). He likes the citrus zing!

2. If you have a craving, walk around, listen to music, and drink water.

3. Eat smaller portions.

4. Replace bread with lettuce (lettuce sandwich).

5. Carry Cinnamon Altoid Mints (0 calories and great for cravings).

6. Weight loss is calories in versus calories out.

A crazy thing happened about two years before our interview when James got Covid and lost his sense of taste and smell. He has never regained it, and it's been helpful because he no longer has cravings. He can sense the citrus zing in lemonade but not the taste.

James shared that early on in his weight loss journey, his trainer said, "You know, if you had not woken up one morning and decided you didn't want to be the fat guy anymore, and you wanted to be a different individual, you do realize that you would probably not be here for your kids' graduations from college, right? You realized time was running out." James encourages anyone who is severely obese to pause for a moment and ask yourself if it's really worth all the extra time you get to spend with your family down the road for that nutty bar or that Coke or whatever it is. Is it worth the moment of joy that you receive from eating that one thing versus a lifetime of joy that you will miss? Instead of focusing on the now, we must focus on the future.

James shared a story of a friend of his who was large like he was before losing weight. James had encouraged his good friend to lose the weight since he was on a one-way journey to an early death. His friend retorted that "James, we all have to die sometime. I might as well die happy!" His friend died in 2022 with gout, diabetes, and cancer at the very end. Now his third grandchild is on the way, and he won't have the joy of meeting her. He had nobody to blame but himself. James stresses that it is necessary to change your mind about your health. You must make a lifestyle change and thoroughly commit to it.

One time during a trip to Las Vegas with his son and friends, they were standing in the lobby of the Bellagio Hotel, and he commented to his son that they looked like all the beautiful people. In the past, he would notice when people pointed at him and made comments or gestures about his large size. Although he still sees himself as "the fat guy", he is excited to no longer be one of the fat guys.

Are you ready to be the best version of yourself? Make the decision, create your plan, and get your body back!

For additional resources, please visit Losing50After50.com.

In the next chapter, you'll hear from Jayme, who lost 148 pounds, gained back 78, then successfully lost 58 pounds and is thriving in maintenance!

CHAPTER 6
JAYME'S STORY

J ayme and I have known each other since high school. I have always known Jayme to be health conscious but also one to battle with her weight. It was so fun interviewing her and realizing that she was winning the battle and had put good habits in place so that she would continue to be on the winning side.

Jayme said she felt like she woke up one day, and spontaneous obesity happened. She is 5'5" and, on her way to 264 pounds, there was no "ah-ha" moment when she realized she had a problem. She was 40 years old and knew she had to do something to drop some weight. She joined Jenny Craig and went from 264 to 116 pounds. While she had success on the diet, she felt like she learned all the tricks to successful weigh-ins instead of a healthy approach to weight loss. After losing weight with the Jenny Craig program, she did not understand maintenance, so she gained back more than half of the weight she had lost. Anyone can follow a program for the short term, but when the program stops, the weight often comes back on.

At age 50, Jayme's weight had gone back up to 194 pounds. Once she created a plan she would live with, she dropped 58 pounds in nine months. Jayme is now down to 136 pounds with a goal of maintaining her weight in the 125–130-pound range. This is the weight where she feels comfortable. She believes a 5-pound range is helpful. Getting education and changing lifelong habits are the keys to keeping the weight off long-term.

Jayme became a professional weight loss coach while working for a couple, where the man was an MMA Fighter and the lady was a nutritionist. They helped their clients with the HCG diet, where they would give themselves shots and keep their calories to between 500-800 per day, eating primarily high protein. She helped her clients with accountability, support, reviewing food journals, and being available by phone.

She shared that weight loss can become an obsession but also a personal failure if you do not lose weight. Everyone has a unique journey. It is not only about calories in versus calories out. The calories from candy bars are different from broccoli. Women have other factors, like hormones.

While she doesn't recommend any specific programs, like Jenny Craig, she feels it's important to keep a food journal and to be honest with yourself. Accountability is extremely important. Log the candy bar and pint of ice cream if you eat it. By using a food journal and weighing daily, you can quickly spot where things went south if your weight is not decreasing. She also strongly suggests taking your measurements and tracking those changes over time. She is a fan of FitBit and feels it can be extremely helpful in reviewing your weight history and tracking your weight and calories.

The mental side of weight loss is the toughest part. You have to know that your body weight will go up and down. Your weight is affected by food, water, workouts, and hormones. If you weigh yourself once a week, do it on the same day and at the same time. However, both Jayme and I feel it is better to weigh daily so that you become accustomed to the fluctuations which occur naturally. When you only weigh yourself once per week, you do not have the benefit of seeing your weight go down during that seven-day interval and seeing the new lower weight. Sometimes we can identify a certain food that made our weight go up from one day to the next. For instance, when I eat sushi, my weight will go up 2 pounds the next morning. I know this because I've seen it happen many times. Armed with this knowledge, I have two choices: 1) don't eat sushi, or 2) don't freak out when my weight increases by 2 pounds the next day. Knowledge is power!

Everybody is unique and will react differently to different foods. It is good to find what works best for you and modify things as you go along. Take a food sensitivity test and learn what foods you are sensitive to and are causing inflammation. I used the test at www.allergytest.co (not dot com).

There were not any foods that Jayme encouraged her clients to stay away from. Her perspective is that if you restrict something, you are just going to want it that much more. Jayme did steer away from prepacked foods. While she hates cooking, she found foods she could eat every day. Costco pre-made chicken and frozen broccoli for the microwave were great options for her. She also loves cauliflower rice.

Jayme's recommendation for managing holidays and special celebrations is to plan ahead. She said that 10 out of 10 times, your family and friends are food pushers. They do not understand your journey, and they think you look fine. But you are the one who must go home and face the scale the next day. Just remember that they are going to eat all the unhealthy foods, go home, sit on the couch, unzip their pants, and feel miserable. Conversely, you're going to go home, feel great and know that you were successful in sticking to your plan. Bring your own food or find what you can eat from what is served. Finally, it is okay to eat a treat or a favorite cookie. And it's better to eat one cookie at the party than to go home and eat seven cookies!

Another way to approach receiving support from your family and friends is to look at it through a different lens. If you had a life-threatening disease and you had to eat certain foods to stay alive, your family and friends would never push unhealthy foods on you. So, think of being overweight as a disease. If you don't get control of your weight, it will inevitably cause multiple diseases in the future. Plan ahead and bring your healthy food with you when you can't eat at home.

When Jayme's clients hit a plateau, she helped them with little tweaks to their plan. She would also encourage a cheat day and have them increase their water intake. She doesn't mean cheating and having a pint of Ben & Jerry's ice cream. Just do something different and jolt your body off the plateau. Your body has muscle memory, and sometimes you must jolt it out of that memory to get it to lose weight again. A good cheat day can reset your body. This is also a perfect time to eat something you really want. However, depending on what you eat, you might not feel great the next day.

Don't wait to begin your weight loss journey on a Monday or the 1st of the month or year. Just start! (As an aside, I ramped up my walking as soon as the doctor cleared me after my surgery. I decided to change my food intake on Monday, June 6, 2022. It was a Monday, but it wasn't the beginning of the month or year. For me, it's better to just begin something rather than making a big deal out of it or waiting until a specific day. After our interview, Jayme shared that she began her most recent weight loss journey on Monday, June 6, 2022. How crazy is that?)

After falling off the wagon, Jayme would allow 5 minutes of self-flogging. After that, she would say, "You've learned your lesson. Tomorrow, I will start fresh." Even if it happens 5 out of 7 days, do not hate yourself over it. Tell yourself you can still do it. You have to forgive yourself and move on. Tomorrow is a new day. The next hour is a new hour. It is important to catch yourself fast. You *know* better, so *do* better.

When her clients had to cook for their families, she would encourage them to make the basics (what her client needed to eat), then cook add-ons for the family (food her client shouldn't be eating). For instance, cook chicken and veggies for yourself, but add mashed potatoes for the family. It is common for families to be overweight. Start by cooking extras for them, but then slowly take away the extras so they can become healthy too.

Prior to gaining the weight back, she wishes she had known how fast it could all spiral out of control. It is vitally important to write down your daily food intake, even in maintenance. If she had been writing down her foods, she could have pinpointed where things went wrong and stopped the weight gain sooner. She wished she had known her body was physically capable of expanding to 264 pounds. Remember, food is for nourishment and not entertainment.

Jayme did not drink alcohol. She treats it like poison. The liver processes alcohol first before it can process anything else. She wants optimal health function, so she does not drink alcohol.

Jayme was on medication for high blood pressure. After losing weight, she came off that medication without any issues. A motivator to get healthy was the experience of losing her father to heart issues at age 67. She also lost her mother to colon cancer at age 82. It is important to know your family's genetics and diseases and live in such a way as to avoid those illnesses. A benefit of weight loss and tracking your body weight daily is that you are aware of the negative changes in your body and can get medical care faster than if you were not paying attention.

While she likes hiking, Jayme thoroughly believes that exercise is a form of punishment. For her, weight loss was 95% food intake and 5% exercise. Intermittent fasting did not work for Jayme. Instead, she had success with eating frequent meals throughout the day, especially after age 50. For everybody else, they think that weight loss is 80% food and 20% exercise. Remember, if you don't put it in your body, your body doesn't have to work it out. Just don't put unhealthy food in to begin with. For exercise, it is important to find something you love doing for the long haul. As important as exercise is, it is more important to figure out your food intake first.

Jayme's weight loss hacks:

1. Call a friend when you feel tempted.
2. Plan ahead! If attending a party, call ahead and ask for a menu of what food will be served. Offer to bring something you can eat to the party.

3. Whatever approach you take to weight loss, it must be sustainable.

4. Drink lemon water first thing every day.

5. Set reminders on your phone to eat every 2-3 hours.

6. Log the foods you eat. Keep a journal.

7. Sleep is important to weight loss. As a rule, a good sleep goal is 6.5 to 8 hours. Figure out how many hours are best for you. Track your sleep through FitBit.

8. Drink plenty of water. Jayme drinks 125 ounces a day.

9. The body has to heal (through sleep) and flush out the bad (with water).

10. Don't wait to begin your diet on a Monday or the 1st of the month or year. Start now!

Jayme feels that the best part of losing weight is the freedom to concentrate on other things in life, things that are important, like family and friends. When you feel good about yourself and your body feels good, you have the energy and are capable of so much more! It sure doesn't hurt that you feel good about how you look in jeans either!

Would you like more energy and the freedom to concentrate on the important things in life? Make the decision, create your plan, and get your body back!

For additional resources, please visit Losing50After50.com.

In the next chapter, you'll hear from John, who played five sports in high school, lacrosse in college, ran 10 miles per day in his adult years, but still managed to find himself at 314 pounds at age 61.

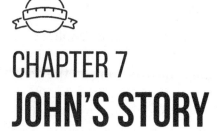

CHAPTER 7
JOHN'S STORY

John is one of my Medicare clients. During the consultation and enrollment, he shared that he had lost a lot of weight in previous years and was on barely any prescriptions.

John is 5'10", and his highest weight was 314 pounds. He was 61 years old when he began his weight loss journey. It took him about three years to drop 95 pounds. He is about 225 pounds now and has a goal to lose an additional 25 pounds.

In college, John played football and weighed 180 pounds. After college, his weight fluctuated, and his high weight was 220 pounds. In order to get the weight off, he took up boxing since it was a great cardio workout. After six months, he was down to 162 pounds, but he felt sick. So, he gained some weight back, and yo-yo dieted over the years. His weight climbed up to 230-240 pounds. Then he changed jobs and put on another 50-60 pounds.

John did not realize his weight had climbed up to 314 pounds. He went for a physical, and his doctor spoke to him about his high weight. John had always been super active, playing five sports in high school, lacrosse in college, and running 10 miles a day in his adult years. He had been working out a lot, eating a lot (at work and home), and felt lethargic, despite still being able to coach his kids' sporting teams (football, basketball, flag football, etc.). For years, his weight fluctuated but usually stayed in the 280-pound range because of his active lifestyle. John's

Achilles heel was drinking 6-8 diet sodas a day and snacking on Hershey's Kisses at his desk at work.

His blood pressure was 125/80 mmHg, his cholesterol was high, and his A1C was greater than 12%. He was on blood pressure and cholesterol medications and knocking on the door of needing an insulin prescription. He decided he did not want to go to doctors regularly and become dependent on insulin. After losing weight, his blood pressure dosage dropped significantly. His blood pressure is now 120/65-70 mmHg with a low-dose prescription. He cut his A1C in half and is now at 6.3%. However, his triglycerides are still on the high side.

John decided to only eat 1,250 calories per day. He decided to eat the same number of calories that his wife ate (and she weighs about 125 pounds). His goal was to lose a pound every week. He began eating healthy food. He limited sodas to once a day if he had any at all. He majorly increased his water consumption.

John also felt that his commitment to intermittent fasting made a difference. Each day, he had coffee around 7 a.m.-8 a.m., breakfast at 9 a.m., lunch at 11:30 a.m. and dinner at 4:00 p.m. His goal was to eat nothing bad after 2:00 p.m., so it had ample time to be digested and used for energy before bedtime. He still had a diet soda sometimes but makes sure to have it before 12:00 p.m.

In place of unhealthy food, he developed a taste for higher quality, real food. He ate all kinds of meat, a favorite being a 6-ounce filet mignon steak with all types of vegetables. For breakfast, his go-to was steel-cut oatmeal with blueberries, skim milk, and brown sugar. For lunch, he would typically eat a sandwich on whole wheat bread (with the crust removed) with one piece of Swiss cheese (instead of multiple slices). For dinner, he would cook whole wheat pasta with homemade sauce, a couple slices of eggplant, and add steamed cauliflower, broccoli, and asparagus. He also drank lots of water with dinner and before bedtime. For dessert, he would eat two ginger snap cookies (just 52 calories). He also stayed away from sauces, salt,

Chinese and Indian food. He eliminated almost all processed food from his diet. He said that processed food was a big part of his weight gain.

For exercise, John began walking the dog 1-1 ½ miles per day, and he did 1-1 ½ hour pool workouts (swimming and walking against the current in the lazy river at a local pool). He also enjoys weightlifting. He used to be a Level B racquetball player, so he likes to break a sweat on the racquetball court. He prefers doing different workouts to break up the monotony.

When hosting or attending social events, John ate smaller portions. For instance, instead of having multiple pieces of pizza while hosting a football-watching party, he chose to only have one slice. He also drank coffee and water and focused on watching the game. At parties, he chose the healthier foods offered (like steak and Brussels sprouts), and he stayed away from drinking alcohol. He avoided potatoes, cheese, and salty dishes. He also chose not to go out with friends if the evening began at 7 p.m. and included food and drinks. He would rather miss the event than put himself in a bad position of eating late in the day.

During his weight loss journey, he enjoyed 1-2 cocktails from time to time. His favorite was Captain & Coke or Crown & Coke. Now, he occasionally enjoys a small glass of red wine at night.

For snacks, John enjoys Greek yogurt, skim or almond milk, and berries in a smoothie. He will split the smoothie with his wife, so it is half as many calories. He also likes raw cashews, apple slices, or dried apricots. He was excited to tell me about a healthy snack of chopped cucumber, chopped tomatoes, and chopped purple onion with Wishbone vinegarette dressing. Although processed, two ginger snap cookies are only 52 calories; they felt like a special treat and were enough. Along with healthy snacks, he said that protein was especially important to his success. He regularly ate chicken, peanut butter, and yogurt. He also shared that he had chicken in the fridge "all the time".

In his excitement about his wife's cooking, he shared a few basic recipes. For pork ribs, they would bake them in a dish on top of a chopped apple and two bags of sour kraut. This would be served with mashed potatoes and beans in small portions. For chili, they would take lean ground beef, add five types of beans and a jar of salsa, and then simmer it in the crock pot. After the chili is made, they freeze small portions and heat them up later for a healthy meal. For a shrimp dish, he uses "Bubbies" horse radish with ketchup as a shrimp cocktail sauce. He also loves a good Jersey Mike's Philly Cheesesteak sandwich and will split it with his wife. He mentioned that his wife makes a tasty scratch vanilla pudding with fruit, and they enjoy small portions.

He shared that his wife was totally committed to healthy eating and cooked healthy recipes regularly. He loves eating her cooking and appreciates her support.

When eating at restaurants, John splits the meal with his wife. He shared that they don't go out to restaurants as much as they used to. If he had a craving for something sweet, he would buy an ice cream cone from Chick-fil-A. Sometimes he would buy a small Mac-N-Cheese and share it with his wife. When they went to KFC (Kentucky Fried Chicken), he would remove the skin from the chicken and eat a small portion of potatoes.

After a stint with Covid during the holidays, he gained 10 pounds but was not deterred by his ability to lose weight. He made a commitment to get back to losing weight after the holidays.

John did not experience any plateaus, as he consistently lost weight with what he was doing. He would weigh himself monthly, with a goal of losing one pound per week. Though he did not write down his weight previously, he said he would like to begin doing that after our interview. He also did not use any apps to track his weight.

Prior to his weight loss journey, John wished he had known how bad the processed food was for him to eat. He wished he hadn't eaten the French fries, onion rings, and milkshakes (sometimes he had two a day). Eating that way makes you want to eat more of the unhealthy food.

John's inward voice around his weight loss journey was a positive one. He would tell himself to get out of bed in the morning and start his day. His goal was to do a little more every day (than he did the day before). He focused on building his leg muscles, knowing that stronger leg muscles would allow him to do a variety of exercises. Regular workouts make you feel great and make you want to do more.

After a day of poor eating, he would eat breakfast the following morning and then decide not to eat again until 3:00 p.m. Since oatmeal gives such great energy and fiber, he rarely skipped breakfast. Because he rarely weighed himself (thereby never showing an increase in weight), he did not have any good or bad self-talk around gaining weight. When he was tempted to eat food he shouldn't eat, he would ask himself if he had eaten anything bad that day and consider the time of day. He shared that the earlier you eat bad foods in the day, the more time you have to burn the calories before bedtime. John eats so clean that when he eats food that he shouldn't, he can feel his body react to it (specifically in his big toe).

John added vitamins to his regimen. He took multi-vitamins, Vitamin C, B-12, Magnesium, Vitamin D each morning, and a hemp gummy (available over the counter) before bed. His skin looks fantastic, and he feels better.

John's weight loss hacks:

1. Use smaller plates and serve smaller portions.
2. Split meals with his wife at home and at restaurants.
3. Always have healthy food in the fridge.
4. Make meals ahead of time and freeze them (so you always have healthy options).
5. Drink lots of water daily (96 ounces), plus coffee. Use filtered water, not bottled. Stay hydrated.
6. Drink Metamucil (fiber) 2-3 times per day.
7. Do not buy anything from the grocery store, which will cause a problem.

8. Use ¼ to ½ of a packet of Country Time strawberry lemonade in 16 ounces of water. If you want a cocktail, add vodka with water and ice.

9. Eat steel-cut oatmeal for breakfast every day.

10. Sleep is the key. If you are not sleeping well, you know you ate something wrong.

11. Eat 5-6 pickle slices/chips every day. It's good for satiation and acts as a body cleanse.

12. Make smaller batches of food.

13. For a small snack, eat a handful of cashews or apricots.

14. For cheese, only eat real Swiss cheese, not overly processed cheese.

15. When he eats apple pie in the afternoon at a favorite restaurant, he skips dinner. His eating hack is "nothing bad after 2 p.m." and "no eating after 4 p.m."

Toward the end of our conversation, John said about weight loss in general, "It's all about you versus you." Isn't that the truth?! Aren't we all our biggest enemies? We can also be our biggest advocates. The decision lies with us. After all, we are the ones who decide what goes into our mouths and how much we exercise. In order to have a successful weight loss journey, we have to get our eating and exercise right. John shared different stories of friends and neighbors who chose an unhealthy lifestyle and how they are in and out of the hospital, using a walker (in their 40s and 50s), and other limiting outcomes. It motivates him to continue his healthy lifestyle.

What's the best part about losing weight? John said he loves feeling comfortable in his own skin. He feels better now when he goes to the beach. He likes to wear 3-4 shirts at a time and said that he no longer feels stuffed into his shirts. He no longer looks like the big fat guy stuffed into his clothes. He can wear jeans and sport coats and feel good about himself when he goes out. He sleeps better, wakes up feeling better, and now he can easily fit into an airplane seat.

John's final thought was, "I don't want to be that guy with big legs, feeling crappy every night. I don't want to be a crungy old man. That's what I don't want to be. I just want to be me."

Do you want to feel comfortable in your own skin? Make the decision, create your plan, and get your body back!

For additional resources, please visit Losing50After50.com.

In the next chapter, you'll hear from Diana, who decided enough was enough when she looked in the mirror and was grossed out by her size. She felt like she wore ugly clothes and decided she didn't want to be an embarrassment to her husband and kids.

CHAPTER 8
DIANA'S STORY

Diana and I are both insurance agents who help people with Medicare. We met at a past insurance company and immediately became friends. She is a lively person with a heart of gold.

Diana began her most recent weight loss journey at age 52 ½ and 204 pounds. She is 5'4". She shared she had previously been as high as 245 pounds and had lost 105 pounds (bringing her down to 140 pounds) but had gained back 65 pounds. It took a little over a year to lose those 65 pounds. Over that period, she would stop and start multiple times. Finally, she told herself, "You've got to do this for yourself, your health, and your family. If you want to eliminate the pain, you've got to be smaller."

When asked what prompted her to lose weight, she said she was depressed when she looked in the mirror. She was grossed out by her size, her clothes were ugly, and she didn't want to be an embarrassment to her kids and husband. Though she had done previous diets, this time was different. Previous fad diets had her eliminating 1 to 3 food groups and stop eating the foods she loved. She recognized that it was not sustainable.

This time, she hired a weight loss coach who helped her with mindset training, meal plans, and simple exercises. She learned eating a piece of cake wasn't a failure and that a small increase in weight was normal. Diana really appreciated the accountability she received from her coach.

Diana did not follow a specific program. Instead, she focused on low-calorie/high-protein foods. The most liberating advice from her coach was, "Eat anything you want. Just stay within 1,200 calories a day." He encouraged her to keep protein high – at about 80-90 grams per day. He taught her that 80% of her food should come from whole foods. It was life-changing for her to eat what she wanted (within the parameters) and know she was not a failure. According to her coach, to lose weight, women should eat around 1,200 calories per day and men should eat around 1,500 calories per day.

One of her previous diets was the HCG diet. She gave herself daily shots of pregnancy hormones, kept her calories at 500 per day and eliminated sugar and dairy. The calorie deprivation was impossible to maintain, and if she ate sugar, it would stop the whole weight loss process for four days. This type of diet, though it works, was completely unsustainable. When she would eat something outside of the diet, she felt horrible about herself for days and felt like a complete failure. Strict and rigid diets are unsustainable.

For a weight loss journey to work, it must be sustainable. You have to ask the question, "Can I do this for the rest of my life?" Or at least, can I do this while I am working to lose weight? Diana's coach taught her that once she reached her weight goal, she needed to do a "reverse diet" where she added in calories slowly. It's not that she was free to go back to all the bad foods that caused her to gain the extra weight (like people do after a fad diet). She just slowly increased her calorie intake until she stopped losing weight.

Diana exercised throughout her journey. She started small, with 20 minutes of cardio seven days a week, and worked up to 40 minutes of exercise 7 days a week. She enjoyed swimming and riding her bike. She also did strength training, usually four different exercises, three days per week.

Diana ate lots of vegetables and some meat. She used MyFitnessPal to track her calories. She didn't eat a lot of fruit but did eat whole grain bread, especially thin-sliced whole grain bread, Lavash bread, and low-carb tortillas. She would make sandwiches with thin-sliced bread and add lunch meat, veggies, and low-calorie dressings.

Diana avoided cookies and cakes. As a binge eater of sweets, she could easily go from one bite to many bites and then end up feeling sick. She learned a trick to only have three bites of something that isn't in your meal plan. Each bite represents something different, with the last bite satisfying the craving. Other than that, she didn't eliminate any food completely.

Diana shared a couple of her favorite recipes. For breakfast, she takes equal parts of yogurt and low-fat cottage cheese (which she whips herself), and adds a little bit of vanilla, oatmeal, and sliced almonds. She mixes these ingredients together, puts them in the fridge overnight, and enjoys them for breakfast the next day. For an evening snack, she blends frozen fruit and pretends it's ice cream. For a snack, she poaches fruit with cinnamon and stevia. She also mixes *Two Good* brand yogurt and sugar-free pre-made Jell-O, getting protein from the yogurt, instead of eating sugary Cool Whip. For her breakfast smoothie, she mixes two cups of spring mix (lettuce), fiber, frozen strawberries, frozen bananas (frozen without the peel), vanilla protein, and stevia. She enjoys what she calls "Protein Ice Cream" by blending strawberries, almond milk, xanthan gum, and stevia (there are recipes available online for exact measurements). She said, "It's fluffy, like Cool Whip." For coffee, she uses four tablespoons almond milk in place of creamer, stevia, and cinnamon. Coffee is necessary! She is not going without coffee!

When traveling, she ate what was available and did not beat herself up about it. Focus on the long game! When at a burger joint, she ate the burger and vegetables without the bread and cheese. At a steak house, she ate steak, a dry baked potato, and steamed veggies. You can also order off the kids' menu for smaller portions. "Enjoy the meal and go on."

Her family was supportive of her weight loss journey. Her husband was a little cranky in the beginning. When she cooked, that's what the family ate and they could make something else if they didn't like it. When her husband cooked, she would either eat what he had prepared or make something else for herself. Over time, her husband's cooking became healthier, and he began cooking things that Diana could eat.

Diana's internal dialogue was healthy due to her coach. She would tell herself, "I'm not a failure. I can eat what I want and it's okay." Your food choices are cumulative, thus one bad day or meal isn't going to ruin it for you. You've got to lift yourself up. When she fell off the wagon (which was about 4-5 times during her journey), she would tell herself to refocus and start again. Decide what you want more: a piece of cake or to be thin? "It's your mindset that will get you through your weight loss journey". "80% of your weight loss will be from diet alone (the food you eat)". After a day of poor eating, she would say, "Every day is a new day to start over. It's okay." When her weight went up, she would say, "It's okay, as it could just be water. It may not be fat. But keep going, it'll come off. Just get back to it." When tempted, she would remind herself that, "Nothing tastes as good as skinny feels." Whether she said that last phrase through tears or screaming, she would repeat it over and over again.

Diana doesn't drink much alcohol anymore. When she does, she leans toward the lighter alcohols, like vodka or rum, with water and Crystal Light. When she knew of an event that was coming up that she wanted to eat more or drink alcohol, she planned for it. She would have less calories the day or days leading up to the event or eat less food on the day of the event. On her son's birthday, she made his favorite cake and enjoyed a healthy slice!

Diana's maintenance strategy began with reverse dieting and slowly increased her daily calorie intake. She shared that the first few pounds that come back after you stop dieting is water weight, not fat. She focused on not eating junk food. She weighed herself every day during her weight loss journey in the beginning but felt that approach didn't work well for her. So, she started weighing herself once a week. She does not weigh herself regularly in maintenance. Her advice is to eat more fruits and vegetables instead of sweets. You need to "change bad habits into better habits."

Through illness, she stopped dieting. But she also stopped eating, so she continued losing weight. When she ate, she ate what she could and did not worry about the calories.

Diana's cholesterol and triglycerides were all within normal ranges after losing the extra weight. At one point, her doctor put her on a statin drug, but she is off that now. Her knees don't hurt, her back doesn't hurt, and she can easily move around on her crutches (after a recent foot surgery). She feels sexy again! She feels like she looks good again and carries herself well, which determines how people see her.

She wished she had known that fad diets are not sustainable. Mindset is everything. She wished she had known the importance of a diet being sustainable over an extended period of time. Her mind, food, and exercise all had to be sustainable to be successful.

Diana's weight loss hacks:

1. Drink lots of water. Guzzle water when you have the munchies.

2. Drink hot water instead of cold water (which signals to your body that you're full).

3. Hot lemon water is good and is a diuretic.

Diana's final thoughts are, "Don't give up on yourself. You can do anything you put your mind to. Get your mind right."

Are you ready to be the best version of yourself? Make the decision, create your plan, and get your body back!

For additional resources, please visit Losing50After50.com.

In the next chapter, you'll hear from Joe, who believes his weight loss of 74 pounds is the reason he's alive today, despite a newly diagnosed heart condition.

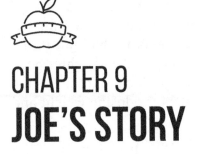

CHAPTER 9
JOE'S STORY

I have known Joe since 2013. He is one of my insurance clients. Joe is a friendly guy who loves helping people and adding value to their lives.

Joe was 65 years old when he began his most recent weight loss journey. He is 5"10, and his beginning weight was 294 pounds. The previous 18 months, prior to our interview, Joe had lost 74 pounds. He was down to 220 pounds with a goal of getting to 200 pounds. Joe mentioned that he would be ecstatic to weigh under 190 pounds since he hadn't weighed that since middle school.

Joe had successfully lost 80 pounds before and kept it off for many years. He did Nutri-System in the 80s and loved their food. It wasn't until his mid-40s that he took a sedentary job where he was driving all the time, eating poorly, and under tremendous stress.

I asked Joe what prompted him to make losing weight a priority. His doctor told him he needed a full hip replacement and had to lose weight prior to surgery. Joe said that for every pound he lost, that represented four pounds of less pressure on his joints. With 74 pounds lost, he now had 296 less pounds of pressure. Wow! Also, recovery and physical therapy would be much easier with a lower body weight.

When questioned about his current approach to weight loss, he said he was on the "Push Away" diet. When eating out at restaurants, he chooses the healthier food on the menu (including no tater tots or fries) and "pushes the food away" once he is full. He often took leftovers home or asked for the meal to be split on the front end and the other half put into a to-go bag. He focused on lower calories overall and lighter beer. This time around, Joe is not using any specific program. He just figured out what worked best for him, began losing weight and continued his new healthy habits.

Joe did not follow a specific workout program. He loves Country & Western dancing, so he naturally exercises doing what he loves. However, as the weight increased, it hurt to dance, especially on his joints. He also loves disc golf, which he hasn't fully returned to yet. Since his full hip replacement and post-operative physical therapy, he is happily doing basic dancing maneuvers and looks forward to having the strength to do the more difficult moves in the future. The brain remembers, but the body is unwilling.

(As an aside, I am currently sitting in an airport while writing this book and waiting for my flight to board. I am sitting at a high-top working table with power outlets. There are four people sitting right across from me eating pizza and drinking beer. None of them are working; they just decided to use the working area as their table. I am so happy I'm not tempted or feeling like I'm missing out. I had an acai berry bowl from Jamba Juice, and I feel full and great!)

Back to Joe, who was not eating pizza... Joe's preferred foods were cereal for breakfast (instead of Sonic or Jack-in-the-Box), a packaged salad once a day (from the grocery store) and a light dinner. He ditched the Frito Lay chips for Kind Bars and Larabars. Overall, he cut down on the volume that he was eating each day. He also consciously chose to stay away from high calorie/low return foods (foods that taste good but have no protein) and high fat/high salt foods, like potato chips and corn chips. He eliminated donuts, pastries, fried pies, and cinnamon sticks from Dominoes 99% of the time. He shared that he allowed those foods 1% of the time. He also added vitamin supplements to his daily regimen.

Joe favored high-quality/low-calorie foods. When he drove for work, he stocked his car with bottled water, Kind Bars and Larabars. He occasionally ate raisins, peanuts, and a small bag of pre-cut carrots. Pre-packaged healthy foods were the easiest, especially when he was feeling lazy. When ordering a hamburger, he would take it with no cheese, extra lettuce, extra tomatoes and sometimes no bun. He enjoyed meats from Mendocino Farms since they were of high quality, like turkey and ham, but with no bread. Since he really enjoyed Nutri-System food, he sometimes included their options in his diet, but not enough to significantly impact his weight loss. He mentioned enjoying their soups, chili, and entrees as a compliment to what he was doing.

While he didn't count his calories or use any apps to track food and exercise, he was aware of what he was eating and monitored himself. Joe likes beer. He shared that he went from Budweiser to Bud Light to Bud 55 to Heineken 00 (which has zero alcohol but also zero taste, according to Joe). Again, with his beer intake, he reduced calories and volume but didn't stop drinking altogether. He drinks 2-3 Bud Lights 2-3 times per week, depending on his calorie intake that day. If he's consumed more calories, he will drink less beer. On occasion, if he's consumed less calories, he'll drink more beers!

When asked how he managed holidays, parties, and restaurants, he mentioned his "Push Away" approach once more. At parties, he either won't go at all (because the temptation was too great) or he stayed away from the food table. At restaurants, he won't order an appetizer and he'll eat 2/3 of the meal and push away the rest or he'll order half to go and only eat half of the meal at the restaurant.

Joe stops eating when he gets sick. This leads to his body burning muscle instead of fat. While it's not healthy to stop eating, it's the way his body deals with illness. After being sick, he put his body on a high protein binge to regain his body mass and to help with recovery.

Joe found that he would hit a plateau when he traveled, especially by eating most meals at restaurants. It didn't bother him, as he just got back on the horse after his trip. Nutri-System taught him that plateaus were normal. To get out of the plateau, he would decrease calorie intake and increase the calories he burned.

While he had considerable support from family and friends, it was a little more challenging with his roommate. They both liked the wrong kinds of foods and snacks. He got around that by making the right foods available, like raisins and Larabars.

There isn't anything that Joe wishes he had known before his weight loss journey, but he shared that it's helpful to set goals around events he'd like to attend. For instance, his son is on one of the Army's sport parachute teams. Joe has a goal to see his son demonstrate at air shows and sporting events.

As he progressed through his weight loss journey, he would weigh-in one time per week and that worked well for him. He kept himself motivated by looking at a picture of himself at 294 pounds. A friend of his found the picture and sent it to him when he was struggling with his weight loss. He would look in the mirror and be so happy that he'd lost a lot of weight since that picture was taken. Then he would encourage himself to keep going.

For maintenance, Joe plans to continue reducing the volume of food consumed. For instance, when he eats pizza, he only has three slices from a 12" pizza instead of eight slices (which was his norm). With a smaller stomach, he eats less at each meal. He drinks lots of water and tries to eat a salad each day.

Joe's dependence on prescription medication decreased as well. His doctor lowered his heart medication. His blood pressure dropped 30-40 points. He would like to get off some of his other medications.

After a day of poor eating, Joe would tell himself, "Hey stupid, what are you doing?" When the weight would go up, he focused on getting back on course, like a ship in a storm. You don't get mad at the wind; you just tweak the direction of the ship. Whenever he was tempted, he would ask himself, "Do I really need that? What am I going to give up (to eat this)? Are these stupid calories or good calories? Could I eat half of it instead of a whole?"

Joe's weight loss hacks:

1. Research the best foods/snacks to eat.
2. Plan your calories based on the needs of your body today and/or tomorrow.
3. Eat calories earlier in the day versus later. If you are planning on a heavy meal, eat it earlier.
4. Choose higher quality food in smaller portions.
5. Order grilled onions instead of onion rings.
6. Keep foods like Kind Bars, Larabars, raisins and water in the car.
7. Have a heavy picture of you handy for motivation.
8. Order half of your food to-go at restaurants.

What's the best thing about losing weight? Buying clothes off the shelf! He shared how, during this last Halloween, he was able to buy a Halloween costume at the store. At Christmas, he fit back into his Santa Claus suit. And he was just five pounds away from being able to wear a favorite fur-lined leather motorcycle jacket from the early 1980s.

One of Joe's final thoughts was that it is easy to get lost and stay miserable, being all tied up in yourself. He is so thankful that his son is living his dream and Joe's here to support him. Joe is looking forward to being a grandfather and being alive to participate in his current and future family's lives and activities.

After our interview, Joe updated me that he had been diagnosed with a heart condition. Thankfully, he already taught himself to consume a high protein/low-calorie diet, which has been easy to maintain. Joe shared that his cardiologist had him remove processed cereal from his diet since it was not good for his heart. He feels that if he had not lost weight in recent years, his new heart condition could have been much worse, if not fatal.

Who needs you to be present in their life? Make the decision, create your plan, and get your body back!

For additional resources, please visit Losing50After50.com.

In the next chapter, you'll hear from Patty, who lost 107 pounds in 15 months and was one of my biggest inspirations for my most successful weight loss journey ever!

CHAPTER 10
PATTY'S STORY

Patty and I have known each other since 2005. We live in the same neighborhood and have been members of our neighborhood ladies' group for years. The entire time I have known Patty, she has been heavy. Since I never heard her complain about her weight, I thought she was fine with it. Something I have learned through this process is that no one is fine with being heavy. Imagine my surprise when I ran into Patty walking one morning and looking much thinner than in times past. I remember catching up with her and, of course, congratulating her on success. Then I asked the same question that everyone asks next, "How did you do it?" She said that she had been walking most mornings and changing the way she ate. She made a point to share that she was not following any certain program or doing anything crazy to lose the weight. Patty became a huge inspiration to me. I literally felt like, "If Patty can do it, I can do it."

Patty is 5'9" and began her weight loss journey when she weighed 264 pounds at age 61. Her goal was to weigh 159 pounds, based on height and weight charts that doctors always refer to. It took her 15 months to lose 107 pounds. She now vacillates between 157-159 pounds. She shared that the last time she weighed 150 pounds, she was in her mid-twenties. Patty believes that she was successful and able to maintain her lower weight because she changed her lifestyle, and she did not do a "diet." It is all about your mindset.

Previously, she had tried losing weight with little success. In her 40s, she counted her macro nutrients (carbs, proteins, fats), took Jazzercise classes, and lost a fair amount of weight. However, with long hours at the office and a sedentary lifestyle, the weight came back. Life got in the way of exercise, and she was focusing on building her career.

For Patty, the Covid-19 pandemic was the precursor to making the decision to lose weight. Life had slowed down and there was more time for introspection. She saw overweight pictures of herself and decided she wanted to be healthier.

At first, she did not know how to go about losing weight, but then she joined the "streetwalkers" (a group of ladies who know each other from our neighborhood ladies' group that walk every morning for exercise). They got their name "the streetwalkers" because for easier conversation, they walk in the streets, side-by-side, instead of using the uneven sidewalks. She recounted our 80-year-old neighbor's comment to Patty, "Better keep up or we'll leave you behind!" In the beginning, it was a struggle; Patty did not have the right shoes or clothes. It took a month of consistent morning walks before she stopped huffing and puffing and repeating "aren't we done yet?" as she made her way through the neighborhood. During that time, she bought walking shoes and Dri-Fit clothing. Now Mondays through Fridays, she walks with the streetwalkers 4-5 days a week for 4 miles in about 65 minutes. On the weekends, she walks 5-8 miles.

What kept her going is that she figured if our 80-year-old neighbor could do it, she could do it! And if another lady in the neighborhood, who had total hip replacement in the 18 months prior, could do it, then Patty could do it! Patty enjoys the lively conversation and free "group therapy" from the walks with friends. She also appreciates the accountability it brings. She does not want to be the one who texts the group and cancels. If she would miss a day or two, the streetwalkers would check on her and make sure she was okay. She also does water aerobics twice a week. These are not simply basic water aerobics; they include weights and interval training.

Patty purchased a FitBit to track her steps. One day, she was looking through the mobile app and realized there was a lot of functionality that she was not using. She decided to begin using the technology in her Fitbit to track more than just her steps including sleep data, heart rate, logging water, and other health metrics. Specifically, she would track calories burned versus calories eaten in real time and throughout the day and make her food choices based on the data.

Her philosophy is that it is all about the calories in versus calories out. Patty shared that, in order to lose a pound, you need to have a deficit of 3,500 calories. She gave herself a daily deficit of 500 calories, thereby accomplishing a weekly deficit of 3,500 calories. (In the interview, she mentioned a 750 daily calorie deficit, but the math worked out to a 500 daily calorie deficit for a weekly deficit of 3,500 calories.) Her weekly goal was to lose 1-1.5 pounds per week, based on it being a safe way to lose weight. We clarified that if FitBit tells her that her daily calorie burn was 2,200 calories and she instituted a 500-calorie deficit, her daily goal would be an intake of 2,200 calories minus the deficit of 500, leaving her 1,700 calories to consume. Patty confirmed that she was not starving through the process. She would eat around 1,700 – 1,800 calories per day, which is plenty of food. Now, she did not leave this to chance, she weighed and measured all her food with a small food scale which she purchased on Amazon for under $30. As an Engineer by trade, she enjoys counting calories, tracking it all and reviewing the various data points in the app.

In terms of what Patty eats, she has not eliminated any specific foods. She loves cooking daily and she loves all food, except for liver and onions. Her goal was to increase healthy foods and continue eating foods she loves. She does not seek out "fat free" or "low fat" foods. The foods she ate included yogurt, lasagna, steaks, hamburgers, sandwiches, oatmeal, fish, and chicken. She struggled to eat an adequate amount of protein, so she would include high protein snacks. Specifically, her snacks included: 1 ounce of almonds, 5 crackers, peanut butter, 1 ounce of cheese, 3 servings of fresh fruit, pretzels (which are salty and crunchy), and an apple. Patty shared that she cut out sweets, which was not that difficult because she prefers salty to sweet. Overall, her goal was not to deprive herself. She ate like a hobbit (her favorite movies are from the Lord of the Rings series) by eating 5-6 small meals a day. She did not do intermittent fasting, and she weighed herself every Friday morning.

Patty would drink alcohol during her weight loss journey only when she had calories to give (i.e., enough calories left over after she had her food for the day). She would enjoy a glass of wine or two. Since she is no longer doing a calorie deficit, she enjoys wine regularly.

When Patty attended parties during her weight loss journey, she allowed herself to increase her calorie intake. On Thanksgiving, she added 3,000 calories to her FitBit calorie count and ate what she wanted. She added 3,000 calories a day for a few days after Thanksgiving, because "leftovers are awesome!" On a trip to Chicago to visit family, she gladly ate the amazing Chicago pizza and White Castle mini burgers. She would not beat herself up over the increased calories or eating food that was not part of her new, healthier lifestyle. After parties, holidays, and trips, she got back to her lower calorie eating habits. She would tell herself that, "it's time to get back to it."

When she experienced a three-week plateau with her weight loss, Patty increased her calorie intake for a week (basically stopping her 500-calorie deficit). That was enough to kickstart her body into losing weight again.

Though her family supported her, they would make comments that she was getting too thin. Patty believed this was because they were not used to seeing her that slim and it was a shocking transformation for everyone else. The last time her weight was this low, she was in her mid-20's. When cooking, she would cook the same food for her family, but add more vegetables. It really was not hard or an issue.

During her weight loss journey, her internal conversation was positive. She would turn sideways in front of a full-length mirror and say, "Wow, this feels good!" She loved the improvements and appreciated the support from the streetwalkers.

After a day of poor eating, she would say "tomorrow's another day start over." When her weight would go up, she would tell herself that she needed to try harder and that the increase could be water weight or a false reading. This did not happen very often, and she was never too concerned about it when it did happen. Since she didn't deprive herself of much, she didn't feel tempted very often. So, there wasn't anything specific she would say to herself around temptation.

Patty shared that she wishes she had lost the weight a long time ago. She asked herself, "Why did I wait so long to make this change?"

Her medications have decreased, because of the weight loss. Her blood pressure medication is a low dose and now she is only taking ½ a pill. Her doctor was literally jumping for joy when he saw her numbers. Her mother is a brittle diabetic, so Patty has been concerned about the potential of her getting diabetes. Although not extremely high before her weight loss, her A1C percentage is low now.

For maintenance, Patty walks almost every day with the streetwalkers and has continued weekly water aerobics classes. Typical routine - she eats a small bowl of Cheerios with milk, and drinks a big glass of water (before and after her walk). After her shower, she enjoys her morning coffee and then logs-in for work. She usually works from 8:30 a.m. to 6 p.m. daily. She prepares her weekly meals on Sunday and eats dinner at 6:30pm.

Patty's weight loss hacks:

1. Do what is good for you. You do you.

2. Make it sustainable. Stay away from trendy weight loss techniques.

3. Listen to your body. Your body will tell you if what you are doing is working.

4. Drink at least 96 ounces of water per day. A high fiber diet with too much roughage can still back you up and make you constipated if you do not consume enough water.

What's the best part about losing weight? Patty feels better and has extra energy! She got rid of nearly all her larger clothes and bought a brand-new wardrobe. When she went shopping, she no longer had to shop in the 1X and 2X department. She could shop in the department with regular-sized clothing. The new, smaller clothes were also cuter and looked better on her. Patty found she could also wear previous favorite and high-quality clothes she kept in the back of the closet for 20 years.

I shared that I recently went through my closet and got rid of a bunch of larger clothing. I singled out the nicer high-quality clothing and put the pieces in a large white trash bag. On the bag, I wrote "oh hell no" because I never want to be able to fit into that clothing again. The bag went into the attic, where it will stay until it is donated to Goodwill. My goal is to never return to those sizes again. Conversely, about five years ago, I went through my closet and donated most of my smaller clothes because I was positive I would never be a smaller size again. There is this one red pantsuit that I am totally bummed I donated. Everyone says, "Just buy a new red pantsuit." It's not that easy, that pantsuit was a one of kind. I will keep my eyes peeled for a fabulous new red pantsuit. In the meantime, I am so happy that I was dead wrong about never being able to lose the weight and returning to a smaller size.

Patty shared that she was able to go hiking on a recent trip to California. She realized a lifelong dream and went ziplining. At this smaller size, she feels it is easier to give back to her community through her volunteer work with STEM programs, especially as a woman in Engineering. Overall, she feels the world has opened up for her. She is happy and has confidence and energy. She stressed that the big picture on weight loss is that it's a lifestyle change. Don't beat yourself up over an extra glass of wine, a piece of cake or scoop of ice cream. Be kind to yourself.

Are you able to accomplish your lifelong dreams? Make the decision, create your plan, and get your body back!

For additional resources, please visit Losing50After50.com.

In the next chapter, you'll hear from Sherri, who used the weight loss program, Optavia, to lose 51 pounds.

CHAPTER 11
SHERRI'S STORY

Sherri is one of my insurance clients. She has a wonderful attitude and stays active.

Sherri was 65 years old when she began her weight loss journey. At 5'5", she weighed 202 pounds. After six months, she weighed 151 pounds and was down 51 pounds.

She got serious about losing weight after her doctor shared that her triglycerides were elevated, and her blood sugar level was close to a pre-diabetic level. Both of her parents had heart issues and she was concerned about her ability to grow old with her grandchildren. The extra weight was hard on her knees, and she just wanted to feel better. Sherri had seen friends and family gain weight and have issues with weight loss surgeries. She knew there were no quick fixes, so she had to do something!

Sherri had done Weight Watchers before and liked the idea of being on a program. She chose to do the Optavia program and appreciated their online Facebook group for support and encouragement. With her level of lower activity, she did the five snacks/fuelings and one meal (protein and vegetables) program. She really liked their pre-measured foods and felt the program was straightforward. She ate no fruit or bread on the program. She also stayed away from sweets and foods high in fat (like donuts).

She did not do much exercise on the program. However, she stuck to the program and lost weight. Now, she loves doing activities at her local senior center, like cardio drumming, chair volleyball and chair exercises. Being at a lower weight, she feels like being more active!

Sherri has definitely shifted her food to healthier options. Her favorite snack is *Two Good* brand yogurt and frozen blueberries. She eats meat including chicken, hamburger, tuna fish and turkey. She can enjoy larger servings of meats which are lower in fat, like 7 ounces of turkey. She uses seasonings without sugar and puts curry on baked chicken. She likes to make cabbage soup in her Instapot. She will cook taco meat with seasoning and add it to her salad (with no cheese). Sherri discovered artichoke heart (heart of palm) pasta with veggies. She also likes cauliflower rice with a little bit of butter, mozzarella cheese, salt, and pepper. For a protein meal, she would scramble four egg whites, plus two eggs. She mentioned that you can Google "100 calorie fuelings" for more ideas.

During her journey, Sherri did not drink alcohol because she was taught that it would turn to sugar in her system and that it took three days to get back into fat-burning mode after drinking alcohol. She rarely drinks alcohol now.

Sherri enjoyed tracking her steps through FitBit. Optavia also has an app that members can use.

When Sherri would attend parties or eat out at restaurants, she would take her food with her. Optavia had a brownie that she really liked, so she would provide her own dessert. She would also eat a salad or from the veggie tray and use 1-2 tablespoons of low-fat dressing. She especially likes Boathouse, which is a brand of dressing with a yogurt base. You can find this product at the store where they sell fresh salads. When eating at a restaurant, she would eat what she wanted and then get back to her diet afterward. It usually took a few days for her body to get back to her weight loss journey, after eating out, so she limited how often she ate at restaurants.

Sherri did not experience any plateaus. She credited this to her sticking closely to her eating plan.

Prior to her weight loss journey, Sherri wished she had known about eating smaller amounts and how often to eat so that she would not have gained so much weight. She also wished she had known about how to make healthy foods taste good.

She was fortunate to have support with her diet from her family. Her kids decided to do the Optavia program too and they were all successful with it. In fact, her son-in-law lost 55 pounds. He is an amputee and can now walk without crutches on smooth surfaces since losing weight.

After a day of poor eating, Sherri would tell herself, "Here we go again, you better behave! You don't want to get back there." When the weight went up, she would say, "Okay, we gotta stop! We can't go back up. I never want to be that weight again!" She would also look at pictures of when she was heavier to motivate her to stay the course. She would remind herself that she could fit in her daughter's clothes and she did not want to go back to the larger-sized clothing. When she was tempted, she would ask herself, "Is it worth it? You'll have to start over again the next day." If she wanted chips, she would look at the serving size and select that exact amount to eat. She wouldn't sit down with a whole bag of chips.

In maintenance, Sherri gained a few pounds. She is working to get back to her goal weight. Her maintenance strategy is to eat every 2-3 hours. She likes the Optavia protein bars, and she has added fruits back into her diet. She also eats boiled eggs, cheese sticks, ten almonds at a time, and has one healthy meal a day.

Sherri's weight loss hacks:

1. Only eat "serving size" for chips, and not the whole bag.
2. Make salads crunchy by adding pepperoncini's (instead of croutons), use Romaine lettuce, and add tomatoes and mozzarella cheese (lower in fat).
3. Have yogurt with frozen blueberries.
4. Choose protein source foods based on energy expenditure needs.

5. Drink 8 cups of water per day.

6. Weigh yourself once a week.

7. Eat every 2 ½ to 3 hours.

The great news is that Sherri is no longer on any regular prescription medications. Her feet do not hurt anymore. She sleeps well and has more energy. Her complexion is better, and she feels great. She also shared that she has almost entirely rid herself of reflux.

Sherri feels that a lot of people want a quick fix when it comes to weight loss. It is better to create better habits. Eat to live, not live to eat. She believes people should do a health program that teaches you how to properly eat, and not diet. The best part of losing weight is feeling great and she has more confidence in herself!

Although most stories in this book are about people who did not use a specific program, like Optavia, I firmly believe Sherri's ability to maintain her weight loss is because she changed her eating habits with real food and healthy recipes. She also began exercising and living a more active life.

Would you like to sleep better, have more energy and have more confidence in yourself? Make the decision, create your plan, and get your body back!

For additional resources, please visit Losing50After50.com.

In the next chapter, you get to hear from me again! I share how writing this book has inspired me and the changes I've made because of what I've learned from everybody's story.

CHAPTER 12
KATIE'S INSPIRATION

I've always thought it odd that Grant Cardone says he writes his books for himself. Presumably, one writes a book for others. However, now that I've written this book, I fully appreciate Grant's comment. This book has motivated and inspired me in so many ways. I learned valuable lessons from the folks I interviewed and have put many new habits in place. The information I learned from the interviews has inspired me to stay on the right track to create a lifestyle (not a diet) that I can do forever. The accountability factor is in play as well. I can't write a book about losing 50 pounds and then go and gain the weight back. I will continue to lead by example and do what's necessary to maintain my new lower weight.

One of the freeing things that stood out to me was that I don't have to attend every party or event. If I feel that I would be putting myself in a bad position where I would be tempted to eat the wrong food or eat late into the evening, I don't have to go. For instance, recently, Bill wanted to go see a three-hour movie at the theater. We just came off four days of hosting family and having lots of unhealthy, high-calorie foods in the house. I had eaten some of that food and my weight went up a few pounds. The last thing I needed was to sit in a movie theater, smelling popcorn that I knew I shouldn't eat. My ability to overcome temptation was low. I just needed a few days to get my eating right and build up my resilience again. We ended up seeing that movie two weeks later and I did great! I brought my healthy snacks and only ate a couple bites of popcorn. Success!

Candi mentioned that your mouth can really taste only the first 3-5 bites of food. Diana shared that three bites of food usually satisfies a craving. When I am eating something high in calories, I often remind myself of this fact and limit how many bites I have. After consuming 3-5 bites, I tell myself I've had enough and move on, just like I did with the movie theater popcorn!

Diana mentioned using MyFitnessPal to track her calories and I began doing the same. Jayme, Russ, and Patty also mentioned the importance of logging your food. I began using MyFitnessPal to log my food. As I mentioned earlier, I could not believe how many calories were in some of my healthy snacks. Based on the information, I chose other foods and smaller quantities and learned what 1,200-1,800 calories per day really looked like.

Jayme mentioned tracking her sleep through FitBit. I owned a FitBit but I wasn't using it. I began using it again and I appreciate the information I'm gleaning from my calories burned and my exercise and sleep patterns. I once had a boss who would say, "If you don't know your numbers, you can't improve your numbers." I couldn't agree more!

James adds ¼ cup of Minute Maid lemonade to his water and he carries Cinnamon Altoids in his pocket. I began doing both hacks and they were awesome! Although I am not someone who needs to flavor my water, I appreciate the zing and lemony flavor from time to time. The mints are especially helpful when I am hungry but unable to eat. I keep Peppermint Altoids in my purse, Spearmint Altoids in my car and Cinnamon Altoids in my office. Obsessed? No. Prepared? Yes!

Doc taught me about BMR (basal metabolic rate) and how to increase it through resistance training. During a conversation at the bagel shop, he mentioned that our largest muscle groups are our thighs and glutes. If we focus on these areas primarily, we can increase our BMR faster and burn more calories while at rest. Based on this, I began doing squats during my morning walk. I now pause at one mile into my walk and do my squats. I began with five squats and steadily added two additional squats every couple of weeks. Currently, I am up to twenty squats. Dr. Mark Taylor, my chiropractor, also encouraged me to do squats versus lunges. Squats are easier on my hips.

Doc also told me about smart scales. I bought the RENPHO Smart Scale and I enjoy analyzing all the data it gives me. It is so gratifying to see your numbers improve across all categories as you lose weight. Specifically, it's been great to see that my bone density numbers are within a healthy range, especially given my age. It was a special day when I moved from the Overweight category to the Normal category in weight.

Russ shared the system for figuring out if you are craving something or if you are actually hungry. On multiple occasions, when I've been hungry, I asked myself if I was craving something salty, crunchy, or sweet. Then I looked at the clock and thought about when I had my last meal. If I wasn't craving something salty, crunchy, or sweet and my last meal was 2 hours prior, I realized that I might not have had enough calories. When I'm craving something salty, crunchy, or sweet, and I've eaten recently, the craving is usually due to being stressed about something. Realizing it's a stress response, I usually choose to drink water, have an Altoid or chew a piece of gum. This little trick has saved me from eating additional calories that I didn't really need or to increase the calorie intake of my next meal.

Multiple people shared about the dreaded plateau. I appreciated the perspective on hitting a plateau and to embrace and celebrate it. When Russ asked if it feels like your bra is falling off, I had to laugh. At that point, my bra was absolutely falling off despite my weight loss stalling. It was good to be reminded that our bodies must adjust to our new lower weight, and this can take time. The weight loss journey is a process that must be understood and respected. Having this knowledge has lessened my frustration with hitting plateaus.

While it seems obvious, Sherri told me that she no longer sits down with a whole bag of chips. Instead, she only serves herself one serving. While I sometimes will still sit down with a bag of chips in my lap (I'm human), I have often incorporated Sherri's approach. I'll stop and count out one serving size of chips and put them in a bowl and then go sit down with my bowl of chips. Sometimes, I'll eat from the bag but count the chips as I go and stop when I hit one serving size. It's especially helpful when I'm tracking my calories and have to log the chips I eat. Logging keeps me accountable to my calorie goals for the day.

I adopted Joe's "Push Away" diet. When I eat in restaurants, I decide ahead of time to eat only half of what I'm served and take the rest to go unless my serving is small to begin with. I also do my best to eat slowly and stop eating when I feel full. I also think about what time of the day I'm eating heavier meals and plan to have those earlier in the day versus later.

John shared about his habit of not having anything bad to eat after 2 p.m. and having dinner around 4 p.m. Although I'll still eat after 4 p.m., I usually try to have my dinner by 6 p.m. This gives my body ample time to burn the calories from dinner before bedtime. I've also made John's chili recipe with beans and salsa. I did it recently while on vacation and it was so easy to make and very tasty! I also incorporated pickles into my diet. They are really yummy, crunchy, salty and have very few to zero calories depending on the brand.

John made an interesting comment at the end of our interview that I've thought about a lot. He said, "It's all about you versus you." I have ruminated on that statement many times and considered what mindsets and habits I needed to change to find success with weight loss. It's not me against the world, my culture, the food establishment, or anything else. I have to master myself, make good choices, and stop making excuses.

Patty's approach to and success with weight loss; consistently walking and eating well, was the catalyst I needed to make my own decision. Because of Patty, I was willing to take another look at my own patterns and make the necessary changes needed to lose weight. If it hadn't been for Patty, I might still weigh over 200 pounds and be quite unhappy with myself. I'm so appreciative of her as a role model and for being a huge inspiration for me.

You can't put a price on how amazing it feels to walk into a store featuring beautiful clothing, select a medium-sized-anything, put it on and have it look fabulous! The dress I'm wearing on the cover of this book was a purchase I made during a business conference in Las Vegas. There was a store in my hotel full of beautiful women's clothing. I was drawn into the store by a gorgeous dark blue bikini on the mannequin in the window. I bought a medium-sized bikini bottom and a size large top (something I've never done in my life). Instead, I've always bought large-sized or extra-large bottoms and a smaller top. I was feeling positive, so I tried on the dress too! Honestly, I couldn't believe they both fit so well. When I returned from my trip and modeled my purchases for Bill, he approved! I decided to wear the dress for the book cover...I am not that brave to wear the bikini for the book cover!

The daily experience of not appearing pregnant (when one isn't pregnant) is unmatched! About ten years ago, Bill and I were out on a date, and we decided to do some shopping after dinner. We walked into a women's clothing store and were met by a twenty-something salesgirl. She took one look at me and asked when I was due. I simply said, "Oh, I'm not pregnant." Instead of apologizing for her mistake, she doubled down and said, "You know, there are exercises you can do to make your stomach flatter." I just smiled, not believing she missed her opportunity to apologize and instead furthered her insult. She continued, "You can do cardio and crunches." Instead of biting her head off and ripping her a new one, I politely said, "Thank you" and walked away. Nobody mistakes me for a pregnant woman these days and I'm really happy about it!

Recently, I was brave enough to wear a bikini at the family pool party. While it was a little scary and uncomfortable, I wanted to celebrate my success and not hide under a bathing suit with lots of material. I know bikinis aren't everybody's thing, but I grew up on the beaches of Southern California and I'm a beach girl through and through. Looking decent in a bikini at age 52 feels like a massive accomplishment to me.

In addition to looking great and feeling wonderful, the positive effects on my health are so exciting. I had no idea that my high weight and poor food choices were causing asthma and elevated cholesterol numbers. Currently, I take no prescription medications and have no chronic health issues. I'm so thankful I was willing to go through this weight loss journey. I believe I've added years and vitality to my life.

As I wind down this book, I must ask, "Have you heard enough to make a decision?" I sure hope so! A healthier, slimmer you is inside, and it wants to get out! Your future self is begging you to begin this journey. Do this for yourself. You deserve a higher quality of life. Your family, kids, grandkids, and friends need you to be healthy and thriving. Your future family, kids, grandkids, and friends need you to be alive and present in their lives. Do it for your loved ones.

Make the decision.

Create your plan.

Reclaim your health and get your body back!

If you haven't taken advantage of my free gift yet, go download the workbook now! It's available on my website at Losing50After50.com.

Please consider leaving me a helpful review on Amazon and on my website. I would really appreciate it, and it will help other people find this book and reclaim their health!

ACKNOWLEDGMENTS

The most important thank you goes to God. He allowed me to hit my lowest of lows, helped me find my way out, and gave me the inspiration and words to write this book. To Him goes all the glory!

A huge thank you to my book contributors: Mark W. Taylor, D.C., Jeffrey Schaffer, M.D., Russ Powell, Candi Emerson, James Winters, Jayme Klimczak, John Zatkos, Diana Mays, Joe Mueller, Patty Rohr, and Sherri Warren. Your life experiences and input are what made this book possible. I am positive that people's lives will be changed for the better because of your stories.

Thank you to my family for your support and encouragement during both my weight loss journey and through the process of writing this book. Specifically, thank you to Bill, Alison, Andrew, Mom, Dad, Laurie, Tim, Adeline, James, Chris, Vashti, Austin, Josh, Corban, Greg, Colson, Misty, Rose, Brian, Mike, Annette, Chris, Alithea, Keith, Lisa, Aunt Dottie, and Robert.

Thank you to my closest friends who went out of their way to make sure I always had healthy food at every gathering and rallied around my weight loss and book-authoring goals. Specifically, thank you to Tracy, Becky, Kelsey, Nikki, and Nicole.

Thank you to my colleagues, who cheered me on every step of the way! Specifically, thank you to Kandice, Paula, Leslie, Marilyn, David, Mimi, Lynn, Melanie, Kathy, Sharon, and Mike.

Thank you to my friends at Einstein's Bagels, who celebrated my weight loss and were excited to hear about my daily book progress. Specifically, thank you to Joe, Chris, Robin, Mark, Tina, Sal, and Kelley.

Finally, thank you to my mentors who believed in me and my ability to set massive goals and see them through to completion. Specifically, thank you to Grant & Elena Cardone, and Brandon & Natalie Dawson.

A sincere thank you to the members of my launch team! This is my first book and I wanted to launch it the right way. They delivered BIG TIME! Thank you to Alison, Angel, Annette, Becky, Bill, Bob, Brandon, Buffy, Candi, Cat, Cathy, Chris, Christine, Christy, Cindy, Claudia, Daniel, Darlene, David, Deb, Debbie, Denise, Diana, Dottie, Elizabeth, Eric, Greg, Heather, James, Janice, Jarrod, Jason, Jayme, Jeff, Jenn, Jessica, John, Jonathan, Jorie, Joe, Juan, Kandice, Kathi, Kathryn, Kathy, Katie, Katrina, Kelsey, Kirsten, Kristen, Kristy, Laurie, Leisa, Leslie, Lisa, Lori, Marilyn, Mark, Matt, Melanie, Meredith, Michael, Michelle, Mike, Mohammad, Monica, Nathan, Nicole, Nikki, Patty, Paula, Penny, Gina, Robin, Ron, Rosie, Russ, Salley, Sharon, Sheila, Shelley, Sherri, Scott, Tamara, Tina, Tracy, Valerie, Vashti, and Victoria.

Thank you to all my social media friends who took the time to comment, share words of encouragement, and give feedback.

AUTHOR BIO

Katie Owen loves books but hates diets and books about diets. After accomplishing what felt impossible, which was losing 50 pounds after the age of 50, she was compelled to write her story and the stories of others who had done the same. While Katie thought she might write a book someday, she never dreamed it would be about weight loss. She hopes her book, *Losing 50 After 50,* inspires millions of people to choose health by creating their own healthy, sustainable lifestyle.

Katie lives in North Texas with her husband and two adult children. Since 2003, Katie has branded herself as the Insurance Gal. She runs an insurance agency, helping overwhelmed, Medicare-eligible people successfully navigate the enrollment process. The agency's mission is to enroll 100,000 clients by 2032. As a gifted teacher and strategist, she helps life and health insurance agents launch and grow their own businesses. Katie's agency website is www.insgal.com.

THANK YOU FOR READING MY BOOK!

It has been my pleasure to bring you this book with real stories of weight loss success.

I would greatly appreciate your feedback and hearing your thoughts.

I will use your input to make future versions of this book better.

Please take two minutes and leave me a helpful review on Amazon.

You can also post your review on my website.

Losing50After50.com/review

Thank you so much!

Katie

Made in the USA
Middletown, DE
13 November 2023

42580399R00060